Screening for Depression and Other Problems in Diabetes

Cathy E. Lloyd • Frans Pouwer • Norbert Hermanns
Editors

Screening for Depression and Other Psychological Problems in Diabetes

A Practical Guide

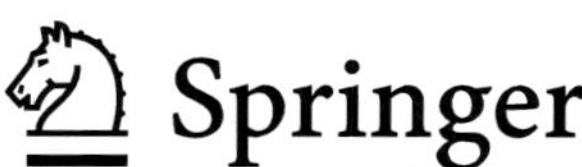

Springer

Editors
Cathy E. Lloyd, Ph.D.
Faculty of Health and Social Care
The Open University
Buckinghamshire
UK

Norbert Hermanns, Ph.D.
Research Institute of Diabetes Academy
Mergentheim, Bad Mergentheim
Germany

Frans Pouwer, Ph.D.
Medical Psychology and Neuropsychology
Center of Research on Psychology
in Somatic diseases (CoRPS) FSW
Tilburg University, Tilburg
The Netherlands

ISBN 978-0-85729-750-1 ISBN 978-0-85729-751-8 (eBook)
DOI 10.1007/978-0-85729-751-8
Springer London Heidelberg New York Dordrecht

Library of Congress Control Number: 2012945541

Printed on acid-free paper

Springer is part of Springer Science+Business Media (www.springer.com)

Foreword

Comorbidity of mental and physical disorders is becoming a major challenge for public health and medical practice. There are several reasons for this including the higher rate of survival of people with chronic illnesses (which increases the number of people at risk for comorbidity), the epidemic increase of incidence of some non-communicable diseases such as diabetes and cancer, and the increasing presence of risk factors (such as physical inactivity) which are implicated in the pathogenesis of several chronic diseases.

The incidence and prevalence of depressive disorders are also on the increase, and depression is today the most frequent mental disorder. It is therefore to be expected that rates of comorbidity of depression and diabetes will grow in parallel to the growth of their prevalence. Yet the prevalence of comorbidity of those two disorders is higher than could be expected on the basis of the increased prevalence of the two disorders. Why this is so remains unclear. There are attempts to explain the higher than expected prevalence, at least partially, by common pathogenesis related to inflammatory processes and immunological reactions and by commonality of certain risk factors, but a definitive answer to the question of high comorbidity rates of depression and diabetes is still lacking.

A factor obscuring the presence of depressive disorders and the growth of their prevalence in people with diabetes is the variety of psychological symptoms that usually accompany chronic illnesses which impose a permanent lifestyle restriction. These symptoms often resemble those of depression, and it is of great practical importance to distinguish them from those of depression because they have to be handled differently.

Health staff in nonpsychiatric general and specialized services often lack the skills and knowledge that would make it possible for them to assess psychological symptoms and their nature. This is the main reason for the fact that a large proportion of depressive disorders occurring in people with chronic diseases including diabetes remain unrecognized and therefore deprived of adequate care. In public health terms, a situation in which a disorder for which effective treatment is available is frequently present but does not get recognized requires the application of screening procedures that will identify persons who are likely to suffer from that disorder.

A number of assessment instruments that could be used to identify individuals likely to be depressed have been produced and used with varying success. Sometimes, their application has been inappropriate because the instruments were not adapted to the cultural or other (e.g., age) characteristics of the group in which they were used. Reports of the usefulness of screening instruments have also varied and sometimes contradict one another.

The volume which Cathy Lloyd and her coeditors have produced, with the help of a number of experts in the fields of psychology, endocrinology, psychiatry, and general practice, is a most welcome answer to questions that have to be answered if we wish to see that screening methods are appropriately used and that people with diabetes in addition to receiving treatment for diabetes also receive support in dealing with their psychological problems as well as therapy for their depressive disorders. I do hope that the book will be widely distributed, translated, and used by many. Its quality and practicability make this highly desirable. Many patients will benefit from this, and the authors of the book chapters will be best rewarded if their work is used and helps to improve the quality of life of people with diabetes and comorbid depression and other psychological problems.

Norman Sartorius

Preface

In recent years, there has been a heightened interest in the psychological well-being of people with diabetes. Current epidemiological evidence suggests that at least one third of people with diabetes suffer from clinically relevant depressive disorders. Furthermore, people with depressive disorders have an increased risk of developing diabetes. This has huge implications for clinical practice as well as for the individual's experience of diabetes. Depression can lead to poor self-care, can affect glycemic control, and can compromise quality of life. Indeed the prognosis of both diabetes and depression – in terms of severity of the disease, complications, treatment resistance, and mortality – as well as the costs to both the individual and society is worse for either disease when they are comorbid than it is when they occur separately. However, in spite of the huge impact of comorbid depression and diabetes on the individual and its importance as a public health problem, questions still remain as to the most appropriate ways of identifying people suffering from depression. Certain screening instruments have been recommended which could be used to identify people who may have depression; however, there are many other tools available and still more tools which have been used in other countries or cultures, in a range of languages. This book aims to provide an up-to-date resource where many of these instruments are discussed, their appropriate use in people with diabetes addressed, and their utility in a range of settings both in the UK and throughout the world examined. This book also considers other psychological problems found to be common in people with diabetes, for example, anxiety, as well as diabetes-specific emotional difficulties such as fear of hypoglycemia. These emotional problems are common; however, to date there has been little practical guidance on how to identify people experiencing these difficulties.

This book is divided into two sections: Part I considers the difficult questions of why, when, and how we should screen for depression and other psychological problems in people with diabetes. The section starts with an introductory chapter by Norbert Hermanns, who considers the reasons why it is important to screen for depression while keeping in mind the limitations of screening as well as the utility. Chapter 2, by Jeffery Gonzalez, moves the discussion on to consider the importance of measuring other psychological problems and how we might distinguish between depression and other forms of emotional distress related to diabetes. In Chapter 3, Richard Holt and Christina van der Feltz-Cornelis take us through the key concepts and principles related to screening for depression. The most common screening tools for measuring depression are then considered in Chapter 4 by Cathy Lloyd and Tapash Roy. Finally in this section, Chapter 5 considers some of the issues related to the cultural relevance of existing depression screening instruments and the implications for practice. Examples from research conducted in South Asians with diabetes living in the UK as well as in Bangladesh are used to contextualize the discussions.

Part II of this book consists of a further five chapters each with a different focus, either on a particular group of people, for example, young people or older people, or a different care setting. The section starts with Chapter 6, by Korey Hood, Diana Naranjo and Katharine Barnard, who show how important it is to ensure that the screening tools used to identify depressive symptoms in young people are appropriate for that age group. The authors also demonstrate the importance of family in identifying psychological problems in children and young people. Looking at the other end of the age spectrum, Chapter 7, by Elizabeth Beverly and Katie Weinger, examines the importance of screening for depression in older people. The following two chapters take a different approach and consider screening for depression in primary and secondary care. In Chapter 8, Margaret Stone and Paramjit Gill discuss how screening for depression in people with diabetes attending their primary care provider can be done, in line with current national and international guidelines. Mirjana Pibernik-Okanović and Dea Ajduković, in Chapter 9, consider the importance of screening for depression in people attending secondary care facilities for their diabetes, where individuals may have the long-term complications of diabetes which may further exacerbate any mental health concerns. The final chapter, written by Frans Pouwer and Evan Atlantis, provides us with a timely reminder of how the concept of depression has evolved over time, and helps us to keep this in mind as we think about the way forward for both research and clinical practice.

Screening for depression and other psychological disorders is important and, as the authors of this book amply demonstrate, is even more vital where people have a comorbid condition such as diabetes. However we still know very little about the effects of screening, both at an individual and a population level. Further research is urgently required in order to clarify this and to ensure that people with co-morbid diabetes and psychological disorders are cared for in the most appropriate manner. We hope that this book helps the reader, be it health care practitioner, service user, or other providers of care, to make sense of the array of tools available for use when identifying those in need of psychological treatment and care. I would like to take this opportunity to extend my heartfelt thanks to all the contributors to this book as well as my fellow editors Norbert Hermanns and Frans Pouwer, for advice and support from Norman Sartorius, and for editorial support from Elektra McDermott and Teresa Dudley.

Cathy E. Lloyd, Ph.D.

About the Authors

Dea Ajduković, M.Sc., is a psychologist at the University Clinic for Diabetes, Endocrinology and Metabolic Diseases of the Merkur University Hospital, Zagreb, Croatia. In addition to practicing health psychology, her professional interests lie in challenges of development and real-life application of scientifically founded educational and psychological treatments for people with chronic illnesses. Dea Ajduković is a research assistant actively involved in the European Foundation for the Study of Diabetes (EFSD) project Does treating subsyndromal depression improve depression- and diabetes-related outcomes? A randomised controlled comparison of psycho-education, physical exercise and treatment as usual. She is currently completing her Ph.D. thesis on the topic of behavioral treatments for depressive symptoms in diabetes.

Evan Atlantis, is a leading expert in mental health, biological and behavioral risk factors for diabetes, and cardiovascular disease research. He completed his undergraduate training in exercise science and doctoral and postdoctoral training in exercise science and epidemiology at The University of Sydney, and was Early Career Research Fellow at The University of Adelaide from 2009 to 2012. He has expertise in evidence synthesis (systematic reviews), epidemiological studies, and randomized trials. He publishes regularly scientific articles that describe the association between clinically significant depression, anxiety or psychological distress, biological and lifestyle risk factors, and chronic diseases. He presents regularly at Australian and international scientific meetings, serves as peer reviewer for more than 30 international scientific journals, and has active research collaborations with groups in Australia and internationally. Dr. Atlantis also leads respiratory disease research in his new role as Senior Research Fellow at the University of Western Sydney."

Katharine Barnard, Ph.D., is a health psychologist at the University of Southampton. She has a long-standing research interest in the psychosocial issues associated with type 1 diabetes in children, adolescents, adults, and other family members. Through her research, she has gained an in-depth understanding of the factors that contribute to quality of life and the impact of diabetes on daily living. The effect of diabetes, both medically and socially in terms of everyday coping, psychosocial impact, and psychological burden, is a multifaceted and complex area, and Dr. Barnard's research to date has made significant advances in the unraveling of these complexities for individuals living with the condition.

Elizabeth A. Beverly is currently a postdoctoral research fellow at the Joslin Diabetes Center and Harvard Medical School. Her research in diabetes and behavioral medicine examines the neuropsychological and psychosocial challenges that arise from following diabetes self-care recommendations and treatment prescriptions. Dr. Beverly graduated from The Pennsylvania State University with a Bachelor of Science degree in 2003 and with a Doctor of Philosophy degree in Biobehavioral Health and Gerontology in 2008. Dr. Beverly regularly participates in research integrating quantitative and qualitative techniques to better understand the management of type 1 and 2 diabetes. Specifically, her research addresses individual patient characteristics and abilities necessary to (1) follow treatment recommendations, (2) improve self-care, and (3) maintain the course of improvements in diabetes self-care and glycemic control. Dr. Beverly has given multiple invited presentations at national and international conferences on the psychosocial and neuropsychological factors that influence the health of adults with diabetes. Further, she has been the recipient of numerous graduate and research training awards.

Sabrina Esbitt, M.A., is a doctoral student in clinical psychology with a health psychology emphasis at the Ferkauf Graduate School of Psychology of Yeshiva University. Her research and clinical work focus on psychological adjustment and self-management in the context of chronic and life-threatening medical illness. She has a particular interest in the role of the family in the development and maintenance of illness beliefs and health behavior. Additional areas of interest include primary care psychology and the integration of mental health care in medical settings. She obtained a Certificate in Public Health from the Center for Public Health Sciences at the Albert Einstein College of Medicine and her B.A. from New York University.

Paramjit Gill (D.M. FRCGP, FHEA) is reader in Primary Care Research at the University of Birmingham and general practitioner in a diverse, challenging inner-city Birmingham practice. His research interests include examining and addressing health inequalities in health and health care, particularly among the migrant communities, and evidence-based health care and its application to health care delivery. He is also the Royal College of General Practitioners Clinical Champion for Social Inclusion.

Jeffrey S. Gonzalez, Ph.D., is a licensed clinical psychologist with specialized training in health psychology. He is currently an assistant professor in the Clinical Psychology Ph.D. (Health Psychology Emphasis) program at the Ferkauf Graduate School of Psychology of Yeshiva University. He is also on the faculty of the Diabetes Research Center and has appointments in the departments of Medicine (Endocrinology) and Epidemiology and Population Health of the Albert Einstein College of Medicine. His research focuses on understanding the role of depression and distress in the management of chronic illness, with a focus on diabetes mellitus. In addition, his research focuses on behavioral intervention research that seeks to improve self-management and distress management in individuals living with chronic illnesses, including type 1 and type 2 diabetes.

Norbert Hermanns, Ph.D., has been the head of the Institute of the Research Institute of the Diabetes Academy Mergentheim (FIDAM) since 1996. He has been an adjunct professor at the University of Bamberg, Germany, since 2007. He has a master's degree in Psychology in 1988 from the University of Bonn, Germany, and was a research fellow from 1988 to 1991 at the Psychology Institute of the University of Bonn completing his doctoral thesis and Ph.D. In 1999, he received his certificate for "Psychological Psychotherapist" and was certified by the German Diabetes Association as a psychodiabetologist. Professor Hermanns is previous chair of the Psychosocial Aspects of Diabetes Study Group (PSAD) of EASD and is a member of BRIDGE, the American Diabetes Association, EASD, and the German Diabetes Association (DDG). His research interests include behavioral modification and weight reduction in people with type 2 diabetes, self-management of people with diabetes, the acute effects of hypoglycemia on cognitive function, treatment of reduced hypoglycemia awareness, and depression and diabetes. He has authored many publications in journals including Diabetologia, Diabetes Care, and Diabetic Medicine.

Richard Holt (M.B. B.Chir., Ph.D., FRCP, FHEA) trained at the University of Cambridge and the London Hospital Medical College and undertook his postgraduate training in diabetes and endocrinology in the South East Thames Region. He was appointed as senior lecturer in Endocrinology & Metabolism at the University of Southampton in May 2000, was promoted to reader in March 2006, and became professor in Diabetes and Endocrinology in September 2008. Richard's current research interests are broadly focused around clinical diabetes and endocrinology and encompass studies of the relationship between mental illness and diabetes. He has published and lectured widely on this subject and has appeared before the UK and European Parliaments to discuss the importance of psychiatric comorbidities in people with diabetes. Richard is currently the European region editor of Diabetic Medicine and reviews editor of Diabetes, Obesity and Metabolism. He is the former chair of the Council of Healthcare Professionals of Diabetes UK.

Korey Hood, Ph.D., is associate professor of Pediatrics at the University of California, San Francisco (UCSF) and staff psychologist at UCSF's Madison Clinical for Pediatric Diabetes. Dr. Hood directs NIH-funded research projects aimed at prevention and treatment of barriers to effective diabetes management such as depression and family factors. He also provides clinical care aimed at promoting health and quality of life outcomes in youth with diabetes and their families. Dr. Hood serves on two national committees for the American Diabetes Association and is on editorial boards for Diabetes Care and the Journal of Pediatric Psychology. Dr. Hood is the author of Type 1 Teens: A Guide to Managing Your Life with Diabetes. His research, clinical care, and service are aimed at helping children and teens with diabetes, and their families, make diabetes a part of their lives while not letting it run their lives.

Cathy E. Lloyd, Ph.D., is an academic and researcher at the Open University, where she is a senior lecturer in the Faculty of Health and Social Care. She has been involved in teaching preregistration nursing and currently teaches health care studies at both undergraduate and postgraduate levels. Her current research interests include the experience of comorbid physical and mental illness, and in particular the impact of the ever increasing burden of diabetes and its psychological sequelae at both the individual and societal levels. Recently, the measurement of psychological well-being and the cultural applicability of existing tools to measure psychological distress in minority ethnic groups has been the focus of her funded research, which has led her to international collaborations with colleagues from the Dialogue on Diabetes and Depression (DDD) as well as from the European Association for the Study of Diabetes (EASD) Psychosocial Aspects of Diabetes Study (PSAD) group. She was honorary secretary of the PSAD and is the current honorary treasurer. She chairs the epidemiology working group of the DDD.

Diana Naranjo is a newly appointed adjunct instructor at University of California, San Francisco (UCSF) in the Division of General Pediatrics. She received her Ph.D. at Arizona State University in December of 2009 in Clinical Psychology with an emphasis on pediatrics. After, Dr. Naranjo completed a year-long fellowship at Children's Hospital/Harvard Medical School where she became interested in working with children and adolescents with diabetes. This past fall, Dr. Naranjo finished a 2-year postdoctoral fellowship at UCSF in the Department of Family and Community Medicine, under the mentorship of Dr. Lawrence Fisher, where she worked on behavioral interventions for young adults with type 2 diabetes. Her research includes an emphasis on bridging the gap for health care services with underserved Latino families, psychosocial interventions addressing depression and distress among patients with diabetes, and the transition between pediatric care and adult care. She currently is working on a research project to better understand the barriers to care for Latino adolescents with type 1 diabetes to help inform a successful transition to adult endocrinology care.

Mirjana Pibernik-Okanović, Ph.D., is a psychologist at the Vuk Vrhovac University Clinic for Diabetes, Endocrinology and Metabolic Diseases in Zagreb, Croatia. Engaged in both the practice of clinical psychology and research on psychological problems in diabetes, she integrates these two sources of knowledge to promote the understanding of psychological needs in people suffering from diabetes. Her professional focus has recently become recognizing subsyndromal depression and exploring treatments which might alleviate its adverse psychological and diabetes-related consequences. Dr. Pibernik-Okanović is a member of the Psychosocial Aspects of Diabetes (PSAD) Study Group of the European Association for the Study of Diabetes and the European Depression in Diabetes (EDID) Research Consortium under the auspices of the Psychosocial Aspects of Diabetes Study Group (PSAD) and European Association for the Study of Diabetes (EASD). She participated in a number of scientific projects, among them multicentric "The development of the World Health Organization Quality of Life Instrument (WHOQoL)." The project was aimed at developing a QoL instrument to be used in different cultural settings. She is currently the principal investigator of the European Foundation for the Study of Diabetes (EFSD) project Does treating subsyndromal depression improve depression- and diabetes-related outcomes? A randomised controlled comparison of psycho-education, physical exercise and treatment as usual.

Frans Pouwer, Ph.D., is professor of Psychosomatic Research in Diabetes at Tilburg University, the Netherlands. His research is embedded within CoRPS, the Center of Research on Psychology in Somatic diseases. He is executive director of the 2-year master of Medical Psychology, Tilburg University. He chairs the Psychosocial Aspects of Diabetes study group of the European Association for the Study of Diabetes (www.psad-easd.eu) and is also chair of the European Depression in Diabetes (EDID) Research Consortium. Professor Frans Pouwer is also a member of the Scientific Advisory board of the Dutch Diabetes Research Foundation.

Tapash Roy (M.B.B.S., D.R.H., M.P.H., Ph.D.) is a multidisciplinary researcher and public health specialist with expertise in the areas of sexual health and rights, public health control of sexually transmitted infections (STIs), comorbid health conditions (depression and diabetes), and the use of evidence in policy making. He is trained in medicine (from Bangladesh) and public health (M.P.H. at the University of Edinburgh, UK) and has a Ph.D. in Sexual Health and Epidemiology from the University of Nottingham, UK. Tapash has worked for most of the past 15 years in South Asia (Bangladesh, Pakistan, and Afghanistan), where he has focused on gathering evidence, informing policy, and building capacity for public health programs. He works closely with national governments (Bangladesh, Afghanistan), as well as with local and international NGOs in South Asia, and academic and research institutions in the UK. Recently, he has been involved in studying the cultural applicability of questionnaires for use in people from minority ethnic groups living in the UK. He has a particular interest in depression and diabetes and has recently completed a systematic review on the use of screening tools for measuring depression in people with diabetes.

Margaret Stone is a nonclinical senior research fellow currently working as part of the Diabetes and Cardiovascular Disease Research Group in the Department of Health Sciences at the University of Leicester, UK. She has worked in a range of health-related topic areas, mainly in primary care settings. Her Ph.D. studies involved a community-based screening program in the field of gastroenterology. For some years, however, her research activities have been focused principally on type 2 diabetes. Margaret is experienced in using both qualitative and quantitative methodologies and also in conducting systematic literature reviews. Particular interests within her recent and current research activities include the development and evaluation of educational interventions, psychological consequences of type 2 diabetes, screening and early detection relating to type 2 diabetes and risk of this condition, perceptions about insulin therapy, and adherence to guidelines. She also has a specific interest in ethnic minority communities, particularly people of South Asian origin living in the UK, who comprise a significant proportion of the local population in Leicester. This interest includes methodological challenges, physiological differences, and diversity relating to beliefs and perceptions.

Molly L. Tanenbaum, M.A., is a doctoral student in Clinical Psychology with a health psychology emphasis at the Ferkauf Graduate School of Psychology of Yeshiva University. She uses qualitative and mixed methods in her research on distress and self-management in diabetes. Her research interests also include relationships between illness identity, understanding and health behaviors, and utilizing expert patient strategies to develop interventions. She has received clinical training in primary care and community mental health settings. She earned her B.A. in Human Biology from Stanford University.

Christina van der Feltz-Cornelis, Ph.D., is a psychiatrist and epidemiologist. She is professor of Social Psychiatry at Tilburg University and director of the Topclinical Centre for Body, Mind and Health of GGz Breburg in Tilburg, the Netherlands. She is director of the Research Program for Diagnosis and Treatment for Mental Disorders at the Trimbos Institute, Utrecht, the Netherlands. She was a member of the Board of the Dutch Psychiatry Association from 2002 to 2005. She was vice-chair of the Multidisciplinary Guideline Working group on Medically Unexplained Physical Symptoms and Somatoform Disorders that was presented in 2011. She was principal investigator of the national Netherlands Depression Initiative from 2006 to 2011, which aimed at improving depression treatment in primary care, general health care, and specialty mental health care settings in the Netherlands. She is cochair of the European Union-funded project "Work Package on Public Health" which aims to develop a research agenda for mental health in Europe. She has (co) authored over 100 publications and supervised Ph.D. students at Tilburg University. Her main research interests are somatic-psychiatric comorbidity, medically unexplained physical symptoms and somatoform disorder, psychiatric consultation models, collaborative care models, and mental health care services research. She is chair of the working group for treatment of depression in diabetes mellitus in the Dialogue on Diabetes and Depression.

Katie Weinger, Ph.D., is an investigator in the Section of Clinical, Behavioral and Outcomes Research and an assistant professor of Psychiatry at Harvard Medical School. She directs the Joslin Diabetes Center's Office of Research Fellow Affairs as well as the Joslin Clinic's Center for Excellence in Diabetes Education. Dr. Weinger earned her undergraduate degree in nursing from Boston College and her doctorate in Human Development and Psychology from Harvard University. She completed postdoctoral fellowships in the Department of Psychiatry at Harvard Medical School and at the Harvard Institute of Nursing Research at Harvard School of Public Health. Her laboratory in behavioral research is funded by grants from the National Institutes of Health, the American Diabetes Association, Harvard Medical School, and several family foundations. Using both quantitative and qualitative methodologies, she studies psychosocial barriers to diabetes care and self-management and interventions that address these barriers. Her areas of interest include affective disorders, distress, and social issues and their impact on diabetes self-care throughout the lifespan.

Contents

Contributors

Dea Ajduković, M.Sc. Clinic for Diabetic Complications, Vuk Vrhovac University Clinic for Diabetes, Merkur Teaching Hospital, Zagreb, Croatia

Evan Atlantis, Ph.D. School of Medicine, Faculty of Health Sciences, The University of Adelaide, Adelaide, SA, Australia

Katharine Barnard, Ph.D. Faculty of Medicine, University of Southampton, Fareham, Hampshire, UK

Elizabeth A. Beverly, Ph.D. Clinic, Behavioral and Outcomes Research, Joslin Diabetes Center, Boston, MA, USA

Harvard Medical School, Boston, MA, USA

Sabrina Ann Esbitt, M.A. Ferkauf Graduate School of Psychology, Yeshiva University, Bronx, NY, USA

Paramjit S. Gill, DM, FRCGP, FHEA Primary Care Clinical Sciences, University of Birmingham, Birmingham, UK

Jeffrey S. Gonzalez, Ph.D. Ferkauf Graduate School of Psychology, Yeshiva University, Bronx, NY, USA

Einstein Diabetes Research Center, Albert Einstein College of Medicine, Bronx, NY, USA

Norbert Hermanns, Ph.D. Research Institute of Diabetes Academy Mergentheim, Bad Mergentheim, Germany

Diabetes Zentrum Mergentheim, Bad Mergentheim, Germany

Richard I.G. Holt, M.A., MB, BChir, Ph.D., FRCP, FHEA Human Development and Health Academic Unit, Faculty of Medicine, University of Southampton, Southampton, Hampshire, UK

Korey K. Hood, Ph.D. Department of Pediatrics, University of California San Francisco, San Francisco, CA, USA

Cathy E. Lloyd, Ph.D. Faculty of Health and Social Care, The Open University, Buckinghamshire, UK

Diana M. Naranjo, Ph.D. Division of General Pediatrics, Department of Pediatrics, University of California San Francisco, San Francisco, CA, USA

Mirjana Pibernik-Okanović, Ph.D. Clinic for Diabetic Complications, Vuk Vrhovac University Clinic for Diabetes, Merkur Teaching Hospital, Zagreb, Croatia

Frans Pouwer, Ph.D. Medical Psychology and Neuropsychology, Center of Research on Psychology in Somatic Diseases (CoRPS) FSW, Tilburg University, Tilburg, The Netherlands

Tapash Roy, MBBS, M.Sc., Ph.D. Division of Social Research in Medicines and Health, School of Pharmacy, The University of Nottingham, Nottingham, UK

Margaret A. Stone, B.A. (Hons), Ph.D. Department of Health Sciences, University of Leicester, Leicester, UK

Molly L. Tanenbaum, M.A. Ferkauf Graduate School of Psychology, Yeshiva University, Bronx, NY, USA

Christina M. Van der Feltz-Cornelis, M.D., Ph.D. Psychology, M.Sc. Epidemiology Faculty of Social Sciences, Tilburg University, Tilburg, The Netherlands

Topclinical Care Center for Body, Mind, and Health, GGz Breburg, Tilburg, The Netherlands

Trimbos Instituut, Utrecht, The Netherlands

Katie Weinger, EdD, RN Clinic, Behavioral and Outcomes Research, Joslin Diabetes Center, Boston, MA, USA

Harvard Medical School, Boston, MA, USA

Part I
What, Why, When and How Should We Screen for Depression?

Chapter 1
Why and When Should We Screen for Depression and Other Psychological Problems?

Norbert Hermanns

Abstract Depression and emotional distress are common in people with diabetes and are major barriers to achieving an optimal quality of life, which is an objective of successful diabetes treatment. Furthermore, emotional distress and depression have a negative impact on the prognosis of diabetes. This chapter reviews the treatment options for diabetes-related distress and considers the screening options for depression and emotional distress with respect to screening performance and acceptability of screening. Screening for emotional problems without a comprehensive management plan has not proven to be efficacious in reducing depression and emotional problems in people with diabetes. Monitoring of well-being is suggested in order to identify people with diabetes suffering from emotional distress and depression. A flow chart depicting a management proposal for patients with emotional problems and depression provides some guidance for clinical care.

Keywords Diabetes • Depression • Emotional distress • Screening • Monitoring of well-being

Introduction

Diabetes is a chronic disease, where short-term as well as long-term outcomes are highly dependent on the successful self-management of the disease. Emotional problems like diabetes-related distress, depressive symptoms, or symptoms of anxiety are common and can be a major barrier to self-care [1–4]. These emotional problems

N. Hermanns, Ph.D.
Research Institute of Diabetes Academy Mergentheim,
Theodor-Klotzbuecher-Str. 12, Bad Mergentheim 97980, Germany

Diabetes Zentrum Mergentheim, Bad Mergentheim, Germany
e-mail: hermanns@diabetes-zentrum.de

C.E. Lloyd et al. (eds.), *Screening for Depression and Other Psychological Problems in Diabetes*,
DOI 10.1007/978-0-85729-751-8_1, © Springer-Verlag London 2013

are associated with reduced quality of life [5], poor self-care behavior [6], worsening of glycemic control [7–9], and a poor prognosis of diabetes with regard to morbidity [10–12] and mortality [13, 14]. Given these negative consequences of emotional problems in diabetes, the presence of emotional problems deserves our attention in clinical care settings.

The good news is that there is also evidence that several treatment options for people with diabetes and emotional problems, especially for depression in diabetes, are available [15]. But unfortunately, emotional problems and depression in people with diabetes often remain unrecognized, making timely diagnosis and intervention difficult.

Given the negative sequelae of emotional problems and depression in diabetes, there are strong and compelling arguments in favor of screening for emotional problems and depression in people with diabetes. Indeed, several clinical guidelines currently recommend depression screening in people with diabetes [16–19]. However, in spite of strong and compelling arguments in favor of screening for emotional problems and depression in diabetes, there are also arguments discouraging the implementation of routine screening procedures. Screening for emotional problems and depression potentially exposes both false positives and true positives (but otherwise unrecognized cases) to stigmatization and potential discrimination by health insurance companies or employers. Thus, the potential benefits of screening for a specific condition have to be balanced against its disadvantages, and in this chapter, this is done by referring to the criteria established by the United Kingdom's National Screening Committee [20]. These criteria refer to the *relevance* of the conditions screened for, the availability of *treatment* options, the *performance of screening tools*, and the *acceptability and efficacy* of the screening program. It will be shown that screening for depression or monitoring of mental health is justified according to these criteria, with evidence provided that depression in people with diabetes is a relevant condition, that treatment option and screening procedures are available, but that the implementation of depression screening needs a structured approach linking screening programs with intervention concepts.

The Size of the Problem

Emotional problems and depression as well as anxiety are common in people with diabetes, whereas other psychiatric disorders like schizophrenia, addiction, or eating disorders seem to be equally prevalent in people with or without diabetes [21, 22]. Thus, this chapter will focus on screening for emotional problems related to diabetes and depression.

Diabetes-Related Distress

Living with diabetes and its treatment demands are often perceived as cumbersome. Worries about late and acute complications, feelings of guilt if getting off the track of the diabetes regimen, and interpersonal problems related to diabetes are frequently reported in people with diabetes. Furthermore, specific treatment options like glucose self-monitoring or insulin therapy are often perceived as a burden especially in people with type 2 diabetes [23–26].

In questionnaires measuring diabetes-related distress like the problem areas in diabetes questionnaire (PAID) or the diabetes-distress scale (DSS), between 12% and 40% of diabetic patients have reported elevated diabetes-related distress. Prevalence rates of severe diabetes-related distress vary according to different countries as well as to different clinical settings [3, 4, 8, 25, 27].

In a longitudinal analysis with 18-month follow-up and three measurement points, 29% of all diabetic patients reported elevated diabetes-related distress at at least one assessment, with 9% reporting persistent elevated diabetes-related distress levels at all three assessments [1]. Thus, severe diabetes-related distress is rather common and shows a great persistence in approximately 10% of people with diabetes.

Research suggests that severe diabetes-related distress and emotional problems associated with diabetes are associated with poor glycemic control [8, 23, 25, 28], which is likely to have a serious impact on the long-term outcome of the disease.

Diabetes-related distress is also highly correlated with elevated depressive symptoms [3, 4, 8, 27, 28]. Since there is evidence that diabetes per se seems to be an independent risk factor for depression [29], it seems reasonable to assume that the risk for depression in people with diabetes is at least partially mediated by diabetes-related distress. However, since the studies demonstrating the association between diabetes-related distress and depression are all cross-sectional, further evidence from longitudinal studies is needed to corroborate this assumption.

In summary, there seems sufficient evidence for taking diabetes-related distress or emotional problems seriously because of the high prevalence and its negative impact on glycemic control and its possible association to depression.

Anxiety

People with diabetes seem to be more frequently affected by elevated symptoms of anxiety [1, 30, 31], whereas findings of a higher prevalence of clinical anxiety disorders in people with diabetes remain controversial [31, 32]. Anxiety symptoms often co-occur with depressive symptoms [30, 31, 33], suggesting that in both symptom groups there may be a more general syndrome of emotional distress in diabetic patients rather than a specific mental disorder like anxiety or major depression. A recent meta-analysis has demonstrated that anxiety or anxiety symptoms show a marginal but statistically significant effect on glycemic control [9]. However, it can be argued as to the extent to which the negative impact of anxiety on glycemic control represents a clinical relevant effect [34].

In summary, anxiety symptoms in people with diabetes appear to be more common than clinically significant levels of anxiety disorders. Anxiety symptoms frequently co-occur with elevated depressive symptoms, thus anxiety symptoms may indicate an elevated level of general emotional distress in people with diabetes rather than be specific for a clinical anxiety disorder.

Depression

In recent years, most research studying emotional problems in people with diabetes has focused on depression or elevated depressive symptoms. This has meant that depression in diabetes is the best understood emotional problem in people with diabetes.

Depression rates in people with diabetes are roughly doubled compared to the general population. A meta-analysis of 42 studies demonstrated that clinical or major depression, based on diagnostic interview and standardized criteria defined by the International Classification of Diseases, 10th Revision (ICD-10) or the Diagnostic and Statistical Manual of Mental Disorders, 4th Edition (DSM-IV), occurred in 11.4% of people with diabetes, whereas the prevalence in nondiabetic people was 5% [2]. People with diabetes also reported more intense depressive symptoms, without fulfilling the criteria for clinical or major depression. Elevated depressive symptoms were reported by 31% of diabetic patients, whereas only 14% of nondiabetic subjects reported elevated depressive symptoms. The doubling of depression rates in people with diabetes compared to nondiabetic people has been confirmed by a more recent meta-analysis [35]. In summary, current evidence shows that approximately every third person with diabetes is likely to report elevated depressive symptoms and more than 10% will suffer from major or clinical depression. Thus, the majority of people with diabetes have a subclinical or mild form of depression, and only a minority have clinically significant major depression.

Since subclinical depression appears to be more strongly associated with poor diabetes outcomes or self-care behavior than clinical or major depression [8], it seems likely that the former might be an indicator of general emotional distress in people with diabetes rather than a necessary precursor of more severe clinical forms of depression [*see also* Chap. 2]. However, independent from the relationship between clinical and subthreshold or mild depression, there is strong empirical evidence that depression in diabetes should be taken seriously. This seems true not only because of the elevated prevalence of depression in diabetes but also because of its negative consequences with regard to quality of life, self-care behavior, glycemic control, complications, and mortality [21, 34].

The Burden of Emotional Problems and Depression in Diabetes

Besides the elevated prevalence of depression in people with diabetes, epidemiological studies suggest that the relationship between depression and diabetes is bidirectional. In other words, there is evidence that depression is a risk factor for developing diabetes [36, 37] as well as for diabetes being associated with a higher risk for depression [37, 38]. Explanations for the elevated diabetes

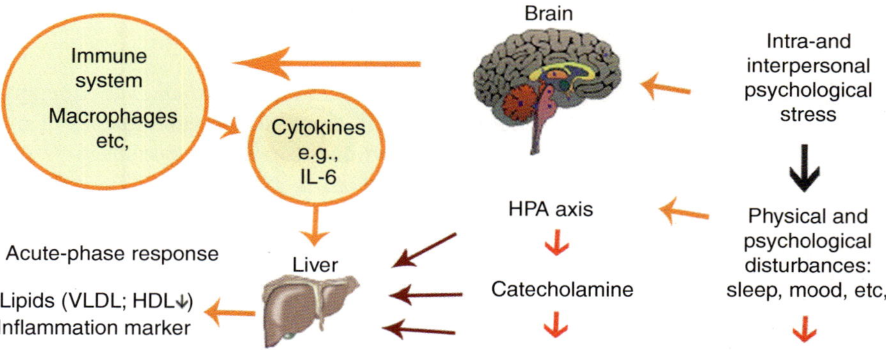

Fig. 1.1 Association between psychological stress, hyperactivity of the HPA axis, inflammatory processes, and reduced insulin sensitivity [40]

risk in depressed people refer mainly to behavioral mechanisms. It is assumed that depressed people might not engage very much in healthy behaviors (e.g., maintaining a healthy diet, reducing overweight, doing regular physical exercise, and adhering to medical treatment), thus causing an elevated risk for diabetes or worsening of metabolic control in diabetic patients. Although at first glance this explanation seems to be plausible, current empirical findings suggest that behavioral mechanisms cannot fully explain this elevated diabetes risk. Prospective studies attenuated but have still shown significant higher diabetes incidence in depressed nondiabetic people compared to nondepressed subjects, even after adjusting for lifestyle factors [37–39]. This may indicate that depression per se is a risk factor for diabetes and may suggest other risk factors like increased levels of inflammation or neuroendocrine hormones [40–42]. Figure 1.1 shows potential links of behavioral and physiological mechanisms in diabetes and depression.

A recent meta-analysis [29] also suggests that diabetes seems to be a significant risk factor for depression, enhancing the risk for depression by 24%. This relationship between diabetes and depression is not exclusively mediated by the presence of diabetes complications [43]; however, it has been demonstrated that the association between diabetes and depression remains significant, even if the multivariate models are adjusted for diabetes complications [38, 44]. This suggests that other factors like diabetes-related distress [4, 8] may be important mechanisms for the incidence of depression in diabetes. Since diabetes per se seems to be an important risk factor for the incidence of depression, the occurrence of depressive symptoms in people with diabetes should be closely monitored.

The relevance of emotional problems and depression in diabetes can be demonstrated with regard to the impact on the prognosis, quality of life, and healthcare costs of diabetic patients, as discussed below.

Reduced Quality of Life

An optimal quality of life is one of the primary objectives of diabetes therapy. However, research has clearly demonstrated that depression impairs quality of life in people with diabetes [5, 45, 46]. In an Australian survey, depression in people with diabetes was associated with poorer quality of life in all eight different quality of life dimensions (physical functioning, role limitations due to impaired physical health, bodily pain, general health, vitality, social functioning, role limitations due to impaired emotional health, and mental health) [5]. The negative impact of the comorbidity of diabetes and depression on quality of life is greater than the sum of diabetes and depression alone, indicating an exponential detrimental effect of depression on quality of life in people with diabetes. Although depression is a rather common condition in chronic diseases [47], a WHO World Health Survey on quality of life in different chronic diseases (arthritis, asthma, angina, and diabetes) showed that quality of life was most impaired in diabetic patients with depression [48].

Self-Care Behavior

Diabetes is a chronic condition for which prognosis is highly dependent on the day-to-day self-care behavior of people suffering from the disease. Behavioral aspects of depression can be frequently characterized by a diminished interest in all or almost all activities and a diminished ability to think or concentrate, or indecisiveness. Thus, it does not come as a surprise that depression in diabetes is often associated with reduced self-care behavior and poor diabetes self-management. A meta-analysis of 47 studies [6] showed that depression was associated with impaired diabetes self-management. There was a negative impact of depression on overall diabetes self-management as well as on specific self-care behaviors such as medication taking, appointment keeping, regular physical exercise, healthy diet, glucose self-monitoring, or diabetes foot care. Ciechanowski et al. showed that there was a linear relationship between the severity of depression and lack of self-care behavior including taking oral antidiabetic medication, less exercise, more unhealthy dietary behavior, and less glucose monitoring [49]. More complex self-care behaviors like achieving and maintaining lifestyle changes were more strongly affected by depression than less complex self-care behaviors like medication taking.

Glycemic Control

In line with reduced self-care behavior, there is strong evidence to suggest that depression in diabetes also negatively affects glycemic control [7]. Studies have shown a significant correlation between depression and poor glycemic control, indicating that depression is a risk factor for poor glycemic control in people with diabetes. However, intervention studies designed to improve depressive symptoms have not always been successful in improving glycemic control [15, 50], indicating that the relationship between depression and glycemic control is more complex than a linear relationship [51].

Late Complications

Since depressed people with diabetes have poorer self-care behavior, it is not surprising that the risk for late complications is higher in depressed people with diabetes than in nondepressed patients. An analysis of research studies based on cross-sectional data concluded that there was a significantly higher risk for sequelae in depressed people with diabetes [10]. This finding was confirmed by more recent cross-sectional findings [31, 43]. However, prospective studies have also been able to show an increase in the risk for late complications in depressed people with diabetes. In a prospective study with 7-year follow-up, Black and colleagues demonstrated that the risk for macrovascular complications was more than three times higher if depressive symptoms were present in diabetic patients at the start of the study [11]. The risk of developing microvascular complications or functional disabilities in diabetic patients with minor depression is increased by a factor of 8.6 or 6.9, respectively. Interestingly, the risk difference for late complications between those with mild and more severe depression was rather small. Thus, it seems that even milder forms of depression have to be taken seriously.

Mortality

An epidemiological analysis of the National Health and Nutrition Examination Survey (NHANES), an ongoing research program to assess the health and nutritional status of adults and children in the United States, also revealed that depression is a risk factor for mortality in diabetic patients, showing that mortality was 54% higher in depressed diabetic patients compared to nondepressed diabetic patients [14]. Furthermore, an elevated mortality risk was only found in depressed people with diabetes and was not observed in depressed people without diabetes. This increased risk for mortality may also differ according to the severity of depressive symptoms. For example, Katon and colleagues have observed a 2.67-fold greater risk in diabetic patients with major depression compared to those with minor depression, although the risk was still increased (by 67%) in the latter group [52]. Interestingly, the relationship between depression and elevated mortality in people with diabetes, although remaining significant, was attenuated by other factors including the presence of late complications and other confounding variables like age, smoking status, overweight, and alcohol consumption. Similarly, Egede et al. also found a significantly increased overall mortality rate in depressed people with diabetes, which was approximately 33% higher than in nondepressed people with diabetes, even after controlling for age, socioeconomic status, lifestyle factors, and overweight [12]. In specific late complications like diabetic foot problems, depression in people with diabetes has been found to be associated with a threefold increase of mortality risk, even when controlling for the presence of macrovascular complications and poor glycemic control [53]. These data indicate further that the increased mortality risk observed in people with comorbid depression and diabetes is not merely a function of lifestyle factors or of a preexisting multimorbidity [13] but that depression per se is an important risk factor for mortality.

Socioeconomic Costs

Depression in diabetes has also socioeconomic implications. People with diabetes and comorbid depression have higher odds of functional disability compared to people with diabetes and no depression [54]. A study by Egede [55] showed that functional disabilities are much more common in depressed diabetic people than in people with depression or diabetes alone.

Depressed people with diabetes are also characterized by an increased use of the healthcare system and 60–80% higher expenditure than in nondepressed people with diabetes [56]. Depression in people with diabetes is associated with increased disability burden, lost productivity, and increased healthcare use and expenditure. In spite of poorer outcome, the costs associated with treatment of depressed diabetic patients are higher than in nondepressed diabetic patients.

In summary, it can be clearly stated that emotional distress and depression in people with diabetes are highly relevant conditions requiring our attention in terms of treatment and care, given the negative impact on quality of life, diabetes self-management, long-term prognosis of diabetes, and elevated health expenditures. Current evidence also suggests that not only clinical or major depression affects people with diabetes negatively but that also mild or subclinical depression, which may also serve as an indicator for general emotional distress, has detrimental effects on quality of life and long-term outcomes of people with diabetes. Fortunately, once depression is recognized, there are a number of treatments available, and it is to these that this chapter now focuses on.

Treatment of Emotional Problems and Depression in Diabetes

Several studies addressed the treatment of depression in diabetic patients. There are different options available for the care and treatment of people with diabetes and emotional problems or depression, including both non-pharmacological and pharmacological interventions, as well as mixed interventions consisting of both pharmacological and psychotherapeutic approaches. In the following section of this chapter, the efficacy of these interventions studied by randomized controlled trials will be summarized.

Unspecific Educational Interventions

Diabetes education has found to be effective in reducing subthreshold depression. For example, Peyrot and Rubin observed a reduction of subthreshold depression 6 months after diabetes education from 38% to 13% [57]. Another study observed reduction of subthreshold depression from 28% to 18% 1 year after diabetes education in a group setting and from 34% to 17% after a diabetes education intervention comprising individual counseling [58]. An interventional study using a behavioral medical education and treatment program for people with diabetes and intensive insulin treatment showed a significant benefit in the reduction of diabetes-related distress compared to a more traditional knowledge-oriented education program [59].

Research has thus demonstrated that diabetes education, providing diabetic patients with skills and knowledge for effective coping with diabetes-related challenges, has the ability to halve the rate of subthreshold depression. These studies suggest that diabetes education enhances knowledge about diabetes and improves coping skills with the challenges of the disease. This could result in a higher perceived control over the course of diabetes as well as in less feelings of being helpless or overwhelmed by the disease.

Psychological and Psychotherapeutic Interventions

Non-pharmacological psychological approaches (e.g., stress management, relaxation and biofeedback, or group therapy) in patients with poor glycemic control showed a significant reduction in anxiety symptoms and depressive symptoms and an increase in psychological well-being [60]. The effect size of these psychological interventions on emotional problems was rather large, whereas the efficacy of these interventions on glycemic control was rather medium sized.

The effect of cognitive behavior therapy in diabetic patients with major depression has been studied by Lustman and colleagues [61]. Cognitive behavior therapy focuses on changing dysfunctional attitudes and negative cognitions of the patient with diabetes and replaces these with more appropriate perspectives and cognitions. In one study, cognitive behavior therapy led to a remission of major depression of 70% but also showed a rather large positive effect on glycemic control [61].

Pharmacological Interventions

In pharmacological interventions, nortriptyline [62], fluoxetine [63, 64], paroxetine [64–66], and sertraline [67–69] were tested as antidepressive drugs in diabetic patients with comorbid depression. The effects of pharmacologic antidepressive medication on glycemic control are rather mixed. Taking nortriptyline was associated with a nonsignificant but negative effect on glycemic control, whereas the other antidepressive medications had a rather beneficial effect on glycosylated hemoglobin.

Furthermore, there are epidemiological [39] as well as interventional studies [70] suggesting that antidepressive medication has a diabetogenic effect per se, pointing to the possibility that the antidepressive effect of antidepressive medication is offsetting the positive effects on glycemic control.

A meta-analysis on the efficacy of antidepressants suggests that antidepressive drugs are rather effective in moderate to severe cases of depression compared to milder forms of depression [71]. Since findings about positive effects of antidepressive drugs are controversial with regard to glycemic control, non-pharmacological approaches for the treatment of depression in diabetes should be the first choice. Furthermore, future studies are needed to determine which substances in which dosage are beneficial in which diabetic patients for the treatment of depression.

Mixed Interventions

In the Pathways study [50] and other collaborative care approaches of the Katon group [72–75], problem-solving treatment or antidepressive drug treatment are used as interventions, with patients having a choice for these specific options. If depression was not sufficiently reduced by the first treatment choice, a switch to the other option or a combination of pharmacological and psychotherapeutic interventions was initiated. The Pathways study showed a large effect on depression but a rather small impact on glycemic control. A collaborative care approach in which metabolic control is also explicitly targeted yielded larger effects on depression as well as on glycemic control.

Effects of Interventions on Depression and on Glycemic Control

In a recent systematic review, van der Feltz-Cornelis and colleagues aimed to establish the effectiveness of antidepressive therapies in patients with diabetes [76]. The authors included 14 randomized controlled trials in their meta-analysis. Figure 1.2 depicts the effect sizes of pharmacological, psychotherapeutic, or mixed approaches on depression severity as well as on glycemic control.

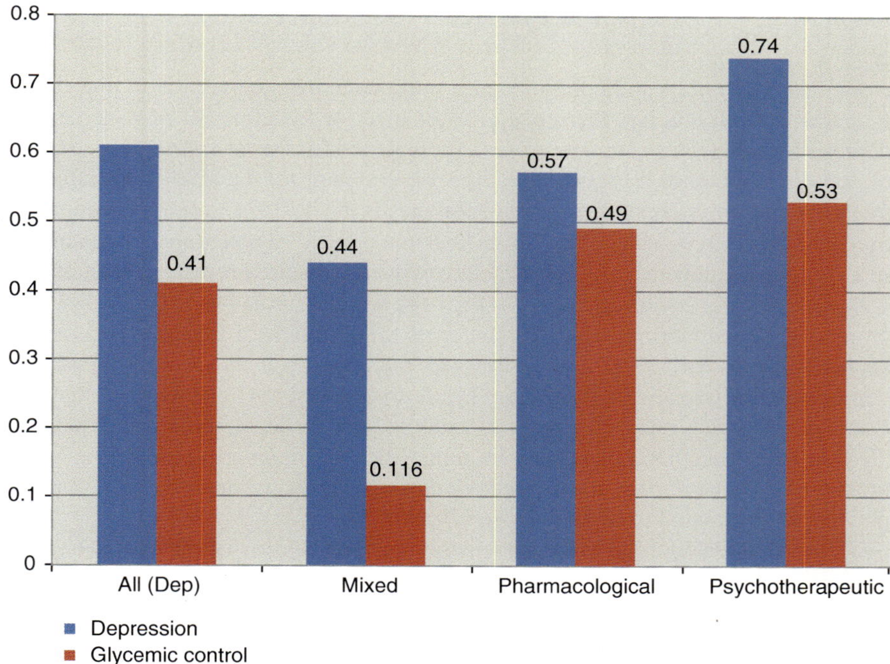

Fig. 1.2 Effects of interventions in diabetic patients with depression [76]

Overall, there are greater effects of antidepressive interventions on depression (severity of depression or depression status) than on glycemic control (glycosylated hemoglobin). The largest effect on depression as well as on glycemic control is shown for psychotherapeutic interventions. Even for pharmacological interventions, only medium effect sizes are reported with larger effects on depression than on glycemic control. But the positive effects on glycemic control rely on a rather small study of Echeverri et al. [69]. In the mixed interventions, depression symptoms are reduced from baseline, but the effects on glycemic control are rather low. There is the possibility that the effect of antidepressive medication, even effective for the reduction of depression, is counteracting the positive effects on glycemic control.

In summary, there are different pharmacological and non-pharmacological interventions available for the treatment of depression in people with diabetes. Applying the second criteria of the United Kingdom's National Screening Committee, the availability of treatment options, the review of the literature clearly shows that screening or monitoring for emotional problems in people with diabetes seems justified with regard to the availability of treatment options.

Screening for Emotional Problems and Depression

Notwithstanding the conflicting evidence outlined above, depression in diabetes is a treatable condition, and there is a great chance for the effective management of depression in diabetes care. However, a prerequisite for this is a timely recognition of depressed mood in diabetic patients. A big problem for the timely and effective treatment of depression in people with diabetes is the difficulties often encountered in identifying depressed people with diabetes in clinical care settings. For example, in a specialized diabetes center of the University of Amsterdam, only 25% of people with diabetes and an elevated depression score were identified by a nurse [77]. In a more specialized German diabetes center, to which diabetic patients with mental health problems are referred, detection rates are up to 56% but still leaving 44% of depressed diabetic patients undetected [4]. A similar result was shown in a study by Katon et al., which reported a detection rate of 51% in depressed diabetic patients [78]. In less specialized diabetes care units, such as in general practice in which most type 2 diabetic patients are treated, detection rates for depression in diabetic patients are estimated to be about 25% [79, 80].

Detection rates for high emotional distress in people with diabetes are also rather low; for example, in a specialized center in the Netherlands, only 29% of patients with elevated diabetes-related problems were identified by specialized nurses [77]. In a German diabetes center, only 18% of patients with high scores on a diabetes-distress scale (PAID) were recognized by a standard clinical assessment done by a physician [4].

The reasons for the low detection rate of depression and emotional distress are multifaceted. Patients seeing a doctor for the treatment of a somatic disease might feel that it is inappropriate to talk about emotional problems like depressed feelings and may report primarily somatic complaints. Also, doctors and nurses may be more oriented towards somatic symptoms of diabetes than emotional problems. Alongside the cognitive symptoms of depression, there are a number of somatic symptoms of depression, which are sometimes confounded with diabetes symptoms, and this will have implications for recognition of depression and treatment of both conditions.

Given the low detection rate of people with diabetes and depression, a regular screening for depression is recommended by several guidelines [16, 19, 81, 82]. A necessary prerequisite for successful screening for depression in people with diabetes is the availability of screening tools. According to the National Screening Committee, screening tools must have sufficient screening performance for identifying depressed people with diabetes but must also be acceptable to the person who screens and to the people who are screened [20].

Screening performance refers to the sensitivity and specificity of the screening tools available. The acceptance of screening refers to the time needed for screening and evaluation of screening tools and the number or percentage of false-positive screened patients. False-positive screened people are usually subjected to (unnecessary) examinations, which in the case of depression diagnosis is a standardized diagnostic interview. This is time consuming and causes extra costs and unnecessary burden. Nonetheless, there are a number of well-validated screening tools available for use in people with diabetes, as the following section outlines.

Screening Performance of Available Screening Tools

One possibility when screening for depression in diabetes is the use of established risk factors for depression. Risk factors for depression are: female gender, living alone, presence of late or acute complications, experience of a critical life event in the past, or poor glycemic control [30, 31, 43]. The screening performance of these risk factors for identifying depressed people with diabetes has not been formally tested yet, however.

Besides the appraisal of risk factors, two verbally asked screening questions have proven to be effective in detecting unrecognized depression in primary care settings [83].

Box

"During the past month have you often been bothered by feeling down, depressed, or hopeless?" and "During the past month have you often been bothered by little interest or pleasure in doing things?"

For a more structured depression screening, there are several validated questionnaires available. In general, all depression scales used to screen for depression or to assess depressive symptoms in the general population could be used in patients with diabetes as well. A recent review about screening tools in diabetes [84] summarizes the screening performance of questionnaires for depression screening in diabetic patients: the Beck Depression Inventory (BDI), the Center of Epidemiological Studies Depression Scale (CES-D), the Patient Health Questionnaire (PHQ 9), and the Zung Self-Rating Depression Scale. The World Health Organization's WHO-5 questionnaire and the PAID questionnaire have also been used successfully for depression screening in diabetic patients [4, 85]. The latter two questionnaires are measuring a broader aspect of negative emotional status in diabetic patients (psychological well-being, diabetes-related distress) than the more specific depression questionnaire.

The screening performance of questionnaires can be evaluated according to their sensitivity and specificity. Table 1.1 summarizes the screening performance for case finding of clinical depression of the above-mentioned screening instruments. There seems to be a general tendency that more specific depression questionnaires show a higher sensitivity and specificity than questionnaires assessing a broader measure

Table 1.1 Screening performance for depression screening in people with diabetes [84]

	Sensitivity (%)	Specificity (%)	Positive predictive value (%)	Negative predictive value (%)
PHQ-9	82	68	53	96
BDI	87	80	47	95
CES-D	85	74	39	97
HADS	77	76	38	95
ZUNG	86	76		
WHO 5	76	48	26	62
PAID	81	74	34	96
Screening questions	97	67	18	99

like psychosocial well-being or diabetes-related distress. The highest sensitivity was reported from the BDI, the CES-D, and the Zung Self-Rating Depression Scale followed by the PHQ-9 and the PAID questionnaire. The specificity of the depression questionnaires is also quite high, ranging from 68% to 80%.

The advantage of a depression screening based on questionnaires is that these are rather easy to administer and to evaluate. Depression questionnaires are not only able to screen for clinical depression but also to identify subthreshold emotional problems.

Questionnaires asking about diabetes-related distress or general well-being might be better accepted by diabetic patients seeking medical treatment because they may expect to be asked about diabetes-related problems or well-being instead of depressed feelings and suicidal intentions. Another advantage is that emotional problems associated with diabetes are brought to the healthcare professionals/the diabetes team. However, this advantage is balanced by a somewhat lower screening performance to detect major or clinical depression of these less depression specific questionnaires.

The relatively smaller screening performance of verbally asked questions may be explained by a varying readiness to speak about emotional problems in diabetic patients if they are directly asked about depressive feelings.

In summary, there are several screening tools with a sufficient screening performance available, ranging from clinical judgment, based on risk factors, over verbally asked screening questions to various questionnaires. For a comprehensive review of screening questionnaires, see Roy et al. [84].

Acceptability of Screening

Besides a sufficient screening performance, screening for depression must also be acceptable to both the patient and the healthcare professional administering the questionnaire. Acceptability refers to the time and effort needed to complete the questionnaires and to score and evaluate the results of these questionnaires. The length of screening questionnaires varies between 5 and 21 items, thus the time required to complete these questionnaires is rather short and is usually less than 5 min. Standardized scoring procedures facilitate the evaluation of the screening questionnaires.

Barriers to screening include illiteracy and the possible cultural unequivalence of the content of questionnaires in different populations and minorities. This is a limitation for the use of questionnaires and needs to be considered depending on the patients being screened.

A major barrier to the application of depression screening is the possibility of false positively screened patients. False-positive screening causes unnecessary diagnostic effort and unnecessary referral, which is time consuming for patients as well as healthcare professionals and is costly for the healthcare system. A low rate of false-positive screening results is therefore an important prerequisite for the acceptability of screening. In Table 1.1, the positive predictive value informs about the percentage of true-positive screened patients. The higher the positive predictive value, the lower is the rate of false-positive screened patients and the higher the acceptability of a screening procedure can be assumed.

As shown in Table 1.1, the positive predictive value of different screening tools varies considerably ranging from 18% of the verbally asked screening questions to 53% for the PHQ-9. Depression questionnaires have higher positive predictive values, indicating fewer false-positive screened patients. Questionnaires measuring diabetes-related distress or general well-being seem less specific and have more false-positive screening results. The low positive predictive values of the verbally asked screening questions are due to the low specificity, since the quality of information obtained from the patient may be highly dependent on the atmosphere in which the questions were asked.

Another problem is that the positive predictive value is highly dependent from the prevalence of a disorder. The mean sensitivity of all screening tools is 84% and the mean specificity is 70%. In Fig. 1.3, the positive predictive value is depicted in dependence from different prevalence rates ranging from 5% to 30%. The lower the prevalence rates, the lower is the positive predictive value and the higher is the number of false-positive screened patients, if a certain sensitivity and specification is given.

In different populations, for example, patients in the outpatient setting of a general practitioner or a clinical population of inpatients with severe comorbidities, the prevalence of depression may vary considerably, yielding different results with regard to positive predictive values and false-positive screened patients.

There are two solutions to increase acceptability of screening by enhancing the positive predictive value, especially in populations with an expected rather low prevalence of depression. In general practice, the cutoff values for the establishment of a positive screening result could be raised. This would result in a higher specificity but at the expense of lower sensitivity. The other solution is a two-stage screening procedure, in which positive screened patients are subjected to a second screening procedure before diagnostic testing is applied or referral to a mental health specialist is done.

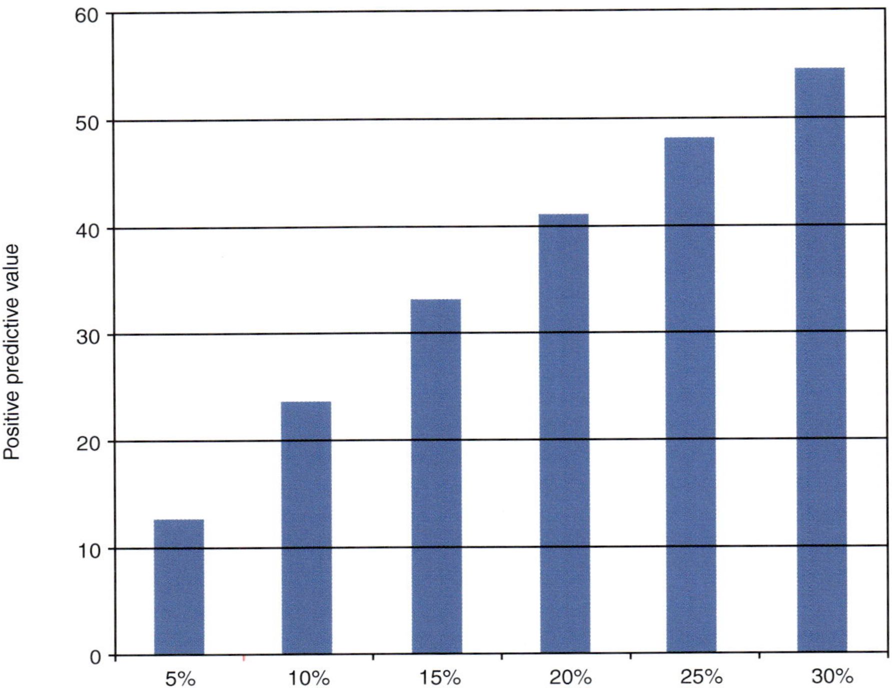

Fig. 1.3 Positive predictive value dependent on prevalence by a given sensitivity (83%) and specificity (70%)

Depression Management in Diabetes Care

Depression management programs for diabetic patients should prove in the long term that they are able to reduce the incidence and prevalence of depression in diabetes and that they are cost-effective [86, 87]. Up to date, there have been no meta-analytic findings based on randomized controlled trials about the effectiveness of depression screening in diabetes. Therefore, we have to rely on a Cochrane review of the efficacy of depression screening in primary care settings [88], where most diabetic patients are treated. The Cochrane review extended the scope of review to the impact of depression screening programs towards the impact on the management of depression in primary care settings. Depression screening is able to identify unrecognized cases, and the Cochrane review reported that screening measures increased the detection rate of depression in primary care settings by approximately 30%. However, depression management in patients participating in screening programs was not significantly better than for the unscreened control groups [88]. Thus, screening without a structured approach for the management of depression seems to have no substantial impact on depression in primary care settings.

The only study examining the impact of screening procedures per se on depression outcomes was conducted by Pouwer et al. [89]. From the 730 diabetic patients participating in a depression screening, 223 patients (30.5%) had an elevated depression score. From these patients, 107 were randomized to a standard care approach (four regular appointments with a medical doctor and/or diabetes nurse without feedback about the result of the screening test) or to an active screening condition (regular medical appointments plus invitation to a diagnostic interview to assess the presence of a clinical mood disorder). If a mood disorder was diagnosed, the treating physician received a letter with the results of the diagnostic testing and a recommendation for treatment of the diagnosed mood disorder. If no mood disorder was diagnosed, the patients received a letter with the results of the diagnostic testing. After 6 months, 70% of the control group and 60% of the intervention group were reassessed. Depression scores showed an improvement in both groups without any difference between the groups. After 6 months, 68% of the control group and 75% of the intervention group still had elevated depressive symptoms [89].

These results seem to indicate, similar to the results of the Cochrane analyses in the general population, that depression screening in diabetic patients without a structured management procedure will not result in a clinically relevant improvement of depression status. Therefore, evidence suggests that successful management of depression in diabetes care settings requires a structured procedure consisting of screening for depression, verification of depression diagnosis, treatment of depression, and evaluation of the treatment response on depression (see Fig. 1.4).

In people with diabetes, the Pathways study is a very promising example of a comprehensive approach to improved management of depression [78]. In this study, diabetic patients were screened for depression using the PHQ-9, and a positive screening result was confirmed using the Hopkins Symptom Checklist. Depressed diabetic patients were offered a choice of antidepressive medication or problem-solving therapy. If depression was persistent after 10–12 weeks, the initial treatment was either intensified or switched (from drugs to problem-solving therapy and vice versa). If depressed diabetic patients did not respond to the intensification or treatment switch, they were referred to a specialized mental health service. This stepped care approach was compared to the control condition in a randomized trial. Members of the control group were informed that they have a depression and were asked to talk to their primary care physician about depression treatment. There was a significant effect in favor of the stepped care approach reducing depression to 40% compared to the control group with a 12% reduction of depression [78].

In summary, this study showed that a structured stepped care approach, containing screening and offering different treatment options and assessment of treatment response, has the potential to reduce depression in diabetes effectively.

In the face of finite healthcare resources, cost-effectiveness of depression screening in diabetes is of course a matter of debate. In the Pathways study, a cost-effectiveness analysis was performed [90]. This analysis shows that within 2 years an increase of additional 61 days without depression per patient was achieved.

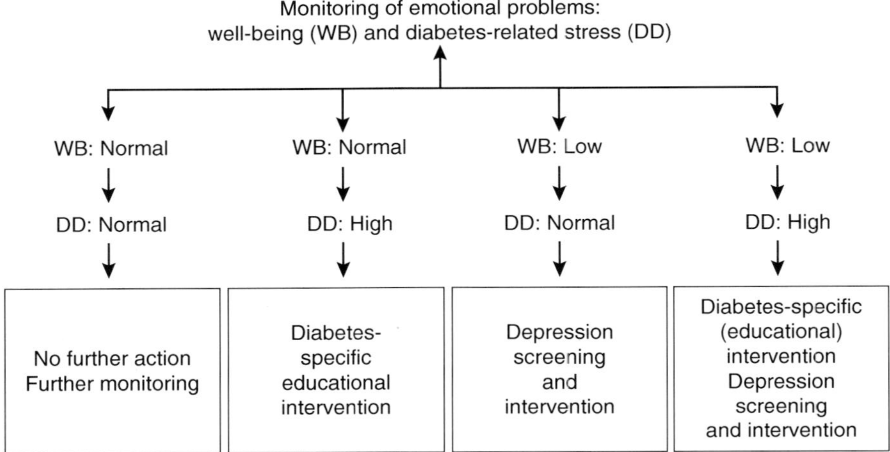

Fig. 1.4 Monitoring of emotional problems in diabetes. Well-being (WB) and diabetes-related distress (DD)

The cost-effectiveness analysis shows that while controlling for various confounding variables, the above-described stepped care approach led to a net cost reduction of 314 USD in total healthcare costs within 2 years.

In summary, there are promising results that implementation of depression screening within a stepped care approach is effective with regard to depression but also with regard to cost-effectiveness.

Practical Recommendations

Emotional problems and depression in people with diabetes have a negative impact on the quality of life as well as on the prognosis of diabetes. Therefore, a timely identification of patients with emotional problems or depression is justified since there are several intervention options ranging from non-pharmacological, educational, and psychotherapeutic approaches to pharmacological treatments. There are also different procedures from the monitoring of well-being and the presence of diabetes-related distress if more formal screening for more severe mental disorders like clinical or major depression is not available.

Monitoring of Well-Being and Diabetes-Related Distress

A study from the Netherlands has demonstrated that monitoring of well-being and diabetes-related distress along with feedback of the monitoring results can lead to a change of routine practice visits with regard to the topics discussed [91]. The study authors reported that discussions were more centered on emotional problems in living with diabetes instead of the technical issues of diabetes treatment. Patients with monitored well-being and diabetes-related distress had similar levels of glycemic control to the control group; however, they made more frequent visits to a mental health specialist and had improved well-being and quality of life scores in a 12-month follow-up [91]. A more recent international study in nine countries (DAWN MIND) has demonstrated that monitoring of well-being and diabetes-related distress along with feedback of the results was able to identify people with diabetes and emotional problems [27]. Those patients with emotional distress were able to improve their general well-being as well as considerably reduce their diabetes-related distress (unpublished data).

Thus, monitoring of well-being and diabetes-related distress along with feedback appears to be a successful method for the routine assessment of emotional problems in diabetes, avoiding stigmatization of patients and aiming at a consensual view of the extent of emotional problems and of possible interventions. Depending on the result of this monitoring, further action can be taken. If diabetes-related problems alone are present, diabetes-specific interventions, for example, change of treatment or problem-specific diabetes education, may be appropriate to solve these problems. If poor well-being is found, a depression screen may be appropriate or at least watchful waiting. The latter means that well-being status should be reassessed if poor well-being persists, and in this case, further action should be taken. If poor well-being and elevated diabetes-related distress are present, it is important to obtain information about the patient's priorities regarding which problem should be addressed first. In populations in which a high prevalence of depression in diabetic patients can be expected, a more specific depression screening using one of the screening tools mentioned in Table 1.1 can be performed.

There is no clear agreement as to the intervals at which monitoring of well-being or diabetes-related distress or a depression screening should be carried out, except that it should be done regularly and at key opportunities [16, 81]. Since depressive symptoms or emotional distress is a risk factor for diabetes, it seems reasonable to monitor or screen for emotional distress at discovery of diabetes. Diabetes is also a risk factor for depression and diabetes-related distress. Thus, it seems also sensible to monitor emotional distress regularly. Experts recommend monitoring emotional distress at least once annually and more frequently if elevated emotional distress is identified [34].

There is also no agreement as to who should monitor emotional distress in people with diabetes. The person who monitors or screens for emotional problems should be capable of giving feedback about the results of the monitoring and should be able to discuss further procedures in an empathic way with the patient. This person could be the medical doctor or a healthcare professional like a diabetes nurse or diabetes educator with communicative skills.

In summary, emotional problems and depression in people with diabetes have a negative impact on diabetes self-care, quality of life, and the long-term prognosis. A timely identification of patients with emotional problems and depression and a structured approach for the management of these problems have proven to be effective in reducing the burden of depression in diabetes. In the short term, healthcare expenditures can be saved. In the long term, a better prognosis, maintenance, or improvement of quality of life can be achieved in diabetic patients, which is the ultimate goal of diabetes therapy.

References

1. Fisher L, Skaff MM, Mullan JT, Arean P, Glasgow R, Masharani U. A longitudinal study of affective and anxiety disorders, depressive affect and diabetes distress in adults with type 2 diabetes. Diabet Med. 2008;25:1096–101.
2. Anderson RJ, Freedland KE, Clouse RE, Lustman PJ. The prevalence of comorbid depression in adults with diabetes: a meta-analysis. Diabetes Care. 2001;24:1069–78.
3. Pouwer F, Skinner TC, Pibernik-Okanovic M, et al. Serious diabetes-specific emotional problems and depression in a Croatian-Dutch-English Survey from the European Depression in Diabetes [EDID] Research Consortium. Diabetes Res Clin Pract. 2005;70:166–73.
4. Hermanns N, Kulzer B, Krichbaum M, Kubiak T, Haak T. How to screen for depression and emotional problems in patients with diabetes: comparison of screening characteristics of depression questionnaires, measurement of diabetes-specific emotional problems and standard clinical assessment. Diabetologia. 2006;49:469–77.
5. Goldney RD, Phillips PJ, Fisher LJ, Wilson DH. Diabetes, depression, and quality of life: a population study. Diabetes Care. 2004;27:1066–70.
6. Gonzalez JS, Peyrot M, McCarl LA, et al. Depression and diabetes treatment nonadherence: a meta-analysis. Diabetes Care. 2008;31:2398–403.
7. Lustman PJ, Anderson RJ, Freedland KE, De Groot M, Carney RM, Clouse RE. Depression and poor glycemic control: a meta-analytic review of the literature. Diabetes Care. 2000;23:934–42.
8. Fisher L, Skaff MM, Mullan JT, et al. Clinical depression versus distress among patients with type 2 diabetes: not just a question of semantics. Diabetes Care. 2007;30:542–8.
9. Anderson RJ, Grigsby AB, Freedland KE, et al. Anxiety and poor glycemic control: a meta-analytic review of the literature. Int J Psychiatry Med. 2002;32:235–47.
10. De Groot M, Anderson RJ, Freedland KE, Clouse RE, Lustman PJ. Association of depression and diabetes complications: a meta-analysis. Psychosom Med. 2001;63:619–30.
11. Black SA, Markides KS, Ray LA. Depression predicts increased incidence of adverse health outcomes in older Mexican Americans with type 2 diabetes. Diabetes Care. 2003;26:2822–8.
12. Egede LE, Nietert PJ, Zheng D. Depression and all-cause and coronary heart disease mortality among adults with and without diabetes. Diabetes Care. 2005;28:1339–45.
13. Katon W, Fan MY, Unutzer J, Taylor J, Pincus H, Schoenbaum M. Depression and diabetes: a potentially lethal combination. J Gen Intern Med. 2008;23:1571–5.
14. Zhang X, Norris SL, Gregg EW, Cheng YJ, Beckles G, Kahn HS. Depressive symptoms and mortality among persons with and without diabetes. Am J Epidemiol. 2005;161:652–60.
15. Petrak F, Herpertz S. Treatment of depression in diabetes: an update. Curr Opin Psychiatry. 2009;22:211–7.
16. IDF Clinical Guidelines Task Force. Global guidelines for type 2 diabetes. Brussels: International Diabetes Federation; 2005.
17. Petrak F, Herpertz S, Albus C, Hirsch A, Kulzer B, Kruse J. Evidence-based guidelines of the German diabetes association – psychosocial factors and diabetes mellitus. J Psychosom Res. 2004;56:672 (Abstract).
18. ADA. Standards of medical care in diabetes – 2008. Diabetes Care. 2008;31:S12–54.
19. Canadian Diabetes Association. Clinical practice guidelines for the prevention and management of diabetes in Canada. Can J Diabetes. 2008;32:S1–201.

20. National Screening Committee. The UK´s National Screening Committee´s criteria for appraising the viability, effectiveness and appropriateness of a screening programme. 2003. www.nsc.nhs.uk/pdfs/criteria.pdf. Accessed 15 Sept 2007. (GENERIC).
21. Petrak F, Herpertz S, Albus C, Hirsch A, Kulzer B, Kruse J. Psychosocial factors and diabetes mellitus: evidence-based treatment guidelines. Curr Diabetes Rev. 2005;1:255–70.
22. Herpertz S, Petrak F, Albus C, Hirsch A, Kruse J, Kulzer B. Psychosoziales und Diabetes mellitus. Evidenzbasierte Diabetes-Leitlinien der Deutsche Diabetes Gesellschaft (DDG) und Deutsches Kollegium Psychosomatische Medizin (DKPM). Diabetes Stoffwechsel. 2003;12:69–94.
23. Polonsky WH, Jacobson A, Anderson BJ, et al. Assessment of diabetes-related-distress. Diabetes Care. 1995;18:754–60.
24. Welch G, Weinger K, Anderson B, Polonsky WH. Responsiveness of the problem areas in diabetes (PAID) questionnaire. Diabet Med. 2003;20:69–72.
25. Snoek FJ, Pouwer F, Welch GW, Polonsky WH. Diabetes related emotional stress in Dutch and US diabetic patients: cross-cultural validity of the problem areas in diabetes scale. Diabetes Care. 2000;23:1305–9.
26. Hermanns N, Kulzer B, Mahr M, Skovlund S, Haak T. Negative attitudes towards insulin treatment in type 2 diabetes seems to be a rather temporal and benign phenomenon: results of an observational longitudinal study. Diabetologia. 2010;53:S380 (Abstract).
27. Snoek FJ, Kersch NY, Eldrup E, et al. Monitoring of individual needs in diabetes (MIND): baseline data from the cross-national diabetes attitudes, wishes, and needs (DAWN) MIND study. Diabetes Care. 2011;34:601–3.
28. Polonsky WH, Fisher L, Earles J, et al. Assessing psychosocial distress in diabetes: development of the diabetes distress scale. Diabetes Care. 2005;28:626–31.
29. Nouwen A, Winkley K, Twisk J, et al. Type 2 diabetes mellitus as a risk factor for the onset of depression: a systematic review and meta-analysis. Diabetologia. 2010;53:2480–6.
30. Peyrot M, Rubin RR. Levels and risks of depression and anxiety symptomatology among diabetic adults. Diabetes Care. 1997;20:585–90.
31. Hermanns N, Kulzer B, Krichbaum M, Kubiak T, Haak T. Affective and anxiety disorders in a German sample of diabetic patients: prevalence, comorbidity and risk factors. Diabet Med. 2005;22:293–300.
32. Grigsby AB, Anderson RJ, Freedland KE, Clouse RE, Lustman PJ. Prevalence of anxiety in adults with diabetes: a systematic review. J Psychosom Res. 2002;53:1053–60.
33. Lloyd CE, Deyer PH, Barnett AH. Prevalence of symptoms of depression and anxiety in a diabetes clinic population. Diabet Med. 2000;17:198–202.
34. Pouwer F. Should we screen for emotional distress in type 2 diabetes mellitus? Nat Rev Endocrinol. 2009;5:665–71.
35. Ali S, Stone MA, Peters JL, Davies MJ, Khunti K. The prevalence of co-morbid depression in adults with type 2 diabetes: a systematic review and meta-analysis. Diabet Med. 2006;23:1165–73.
36. Knol MJ, Twisk JW, Beekman AT, Heine RJ, Snoek FJ, Pouwer F. Depression as a risk factor for the onset of type 2 diabetes mellitus. A meta-analysis. Diabetologia. 2006;49:837–45.
37. Golden SH, Lazo M, Carnethon M, et al. Examining a bidirectional association between depressive symptoms and diabetes. JAMA. 2008;299:2751–9.
38. Mezuk B, Eaton WW, Albrecht S, Golden SH. Depression and type 2 diabetes over the lifespan: a meta-analysis. Diabetes Care. 2008;31:2383–90.
39. Pan A, Lucas M, Sun Q, et al. Bidirectional association between depression and type 2 diabetes mellitus in women. Arch Intern Med. 2010;170:1884–91.
40. Pickup JC. Inflammation and activated innate immunity in the pathogenesis of type 2 diabetes. Diabetes Care. 2004;27:813–23.
41. Howren MB, Lamkin DM, Suls J. Associations of depression with C-reactive protein, IL-1, and IL-6: a meta-analysis. Psychosom Med. 2009;71:171–86.
42. Golden SH. A review of the evidence for a neuroendocrine link between stress, depression and diabetes mellitus. Curr Diabetes Rev. 2007;3:252–9.

43. Pouwer F, Beekman ATF, Nijpels G, et al. Rates and risks for co-morbid depression in patients with type 2 diabetes mellitus: results of a community based study. Diabetologia. 2003;46:892–8.
44. Golden SH, Mezuk B. The association of depressive symptoms with prediabetes versus diagnosed diabetes: is ignorance really bliss? Phys Sportsmed. 2009;37:143–5.
45. Ali S, Stone M, Skinner TC, Robertson N, Davies M, Khunti K. The association between depression and health-related quality of life in people with type 2 diabetes: a systematic literature review. Diabetes Metab Res Rev. 2010;26:75–89.
46. Welch GW, Jacobson AM, Polonsky WH. The problem areas in diabetes scale. An evaluation of its clinical utility. Diabetes Care. 1997;20:760–6.
47. National Institute for Health and Clinical Excellence. Depression in adults with a chronic physical health problem: treatment and management. 2009. http://www.nice.org.uk/nicemedia/pdf/CG91NICEGuideline.pdf. Accessed 12 Mar 2012.
48. Moussavi S, Chatterji S, Verdes E, Tandon A, Patel V, Ustun B. Depression, chronic diseases, and decrements in health: results from the World Health Surveys. Lancet. 2007;370:851–8.
49. Ciechanowski PS, Katon WJ, Russo JE. Depression and diabetes: impact of depressive symptoms on adherence, function, and costs. Arch Intern Med. 2000;160:3278–85.
50. Katon WJ, Von KM, Lin EH, et al. The pathways study: a randomized trial of collaborative care in patients with diabetes and depression. Arch Gen Psychiatry. 2004;61:1042–9.
51. Katon W, Russo J, Lin EH, et al. Diabetes and poor disease control: is comorbid depression associated with poor medication adherence or lack of treatment intensification? Psychosom Med. 2009;71:965–72.
52. Katon WJ, Rutter C, Simon G, et al. The association of comorbid depression with mortality in patients with type 2 diabetes. Diabetes Care. 2005;28:2668–72.
53. Ismail K, Winkley K, Stahl D, Chalder T, Edmonds M. A cohort study of people with diabetes and their first foot ulcer: the role of depression on mortality. Diabetes Care. 2007;30:1473–9.
54. Von Korff M, Katon W, Lin EH, et al. Work disability among individuals with diabetes. Diabetes Care. 2005;28:1326–32.
55. Egede LE. Effects of depression on work loss and disability bed days in individuals with diabetes. Diabetes Care. 2004;27:1751–3.
56. Egede LE, Zheng D, Simpson K. Comorbid depression is associated with increased health care use and expenditures in individuals with diabetes. Diabetes Care. 2002;25:464–70.
57. Peyrot M, Rubin RR. Persistence of depressive symptoms in diabetic adults. Diabetes Care. 1999;22:448–52.
58. Hermanns N, Kulzer B, Kubiak T, Haak T. Course of depression in type 2 diabetes. Diabetes. 2004;53:16A (Abstract).
59. Hermanns N, Kulzer B, Maier B, Mahr M, Haak T. The effect of an education programme (MEDIAS 2 ICT) involving intensive insulin treatment for people with type 2 diabetes. Patient Educ Couns. 2012;86:226–32. Epub 28 Jun 2011.
60. Ismail K, Winkley K, Rabe-Hesketh S. Systematic review and meta-analysis of randomised controlled trials of psychological interventions to improve glycaemic control in patients with type 2 diabetes. Lancet. 2004;363:1589–97.
61. Lustman PJ, Griffith LS, Freedland KE, Kissel SS, Clouse RE. Cognitive behavior therapy for depression in type 2 diabetes mellitus: a randomized, controlled trial. Ann Intern Med. 1998;129:613–21.
62. Lustman PJ, Griffith LS, Clouse RE, et al. Effects of nortriptyline on depression and glycemic control in diabetes: results of a double-blind, placebo-controlled trial. Psychosom Med. 1997;59:241–50.
63. Lustman PJ, Freedland KE, Griffith LS, Clouse RE. Fluoxetine for depression in diabetes: a randomized double-blind placebo-controlled trial. Diabetes Care. 2000;23:618–23.
64. Gülseren L, Gülseren S, Hekimsoy Z, Mete L. Comparison of fluoxetine and paroxetine in type II diabetes mellitus patients. Arch Med Res. 2005;36:159–65.
65. Paile-Hyvarinen M, Wahlbeck K, Eriksson J. Quality of life and metabolic status in mildly depressed women with type 2 diabetes treated with paroxetine: a single-blind randomised placebo controlled trial. BMC Fam Pract. 2003;4:7.

66. Paile-Hyvarinen M, Wahlbeck K, Eriksson J. Quality of life and metabolic status in mildly depressed patients with type 2 diabetes treated with paroxetine: a double-blind randomised placebo controlled 6-month trial. BMC Fam Pract. 2007;8:34.
67. Lustman PJ, Clouse RE, Nix BD, et al. Sertraline for prevention of depression recurrence in diabetes mellitus: a randomized, double-blind, placebo-controlled trial. Arch Gen Psychiatry. 2006;63:521–9.
68. Williams MM, Clouse RE, Nix BD, et al. Efficacy of sertraline in prevention of depression recurrence in older versus younger adults with diabetes. Diabetes Care. 2007;30:801–6.
69. Echeverry D, Duran P, Bonds C, Lee M, Davidson MB. Effect of pharmacological treatment of depression on A1C and quality of life in low-income Hispanics and African Americans with diabetes: a randomized, double-blind, placebo-controlled trial. Diabetes Care. 2009;32: 2156–60.
70. Rubin RR, Ma Y, Marrero DG, et al. Elevated depression symptoms, antidepressant medicine use, and risk of developing diabetes during the diabetes prevention program. Diabetes Care. 2008;31:420–6.
71. Kirsch I, Deacon BJ, Huedo-Medina TB, Scoboria A, Moore TJ, Johnson BT. Initial severity and antidepressant benefits: a meta-analysis of data submitted to the Food and Drug Administration. PLoS Med. 2008;5:e45.
72. Ell K, Aranda MP, Xie B, Lee PJ, Chou CP. Collaborative depression treatment in older and younger adults with physical illness: pooled comparative analysis of three randomized clinical trials. Am J Geriatr Psychiatry. 2010;18:520–30.
73. Ell K, Katon W, Xie B, et al. One-year postcollaborative depression care trial outcomes among predominantly Hispanic diabetes safety net patients. Gen Hosp Psychiatry. 2011;33:436–42.
74. Williams Jr JW, Katon W, Lin EH, et al. The effectiveness of depression care management on diabetes-related outcomes in older patients. Ann Intern Med. 2004;140:1015–24.
75. Katon WJ, Lin EHB, Von Korff M, et al. Collaborative care for patients with depression and chronic illnesses. N Engl J Med. 2010;363:2611–20.
76. van der Feltz-Cornelis CM, Nuyen J, Stoop C, et al. Effect of interventions for major depressive disorder and significant depressive symptoms in patients with diabetes mellitus: a systematic review and meta-analysis. Gen Hosp Psychiatry. 2010;32:380–95.
77. Pouwer F, Beekman AT, Lubach C, Snoek FJ. Nurses' recognition and registration of depression, anxiety and diabetes-specific emotional problems in outpatients with diabetes mellitus. Patient Educ Couns. 2006;60:235–40.
78. Katon WJ, Simon G, Russo J, et al. Quality of depression care in a population-based sample of patients with diabetes and major depression. Med Care. 2004;42:1222–9.
79. AHCPR Depression Guideline Panel. Depression in Primary Care: Volume 2. Treatment of Major Depression. Clinical Practice Guideline, Number 5. Rockville, MD.U.S. Department of Health and Human Services, Public Health Service, Agency for Health Care Policy and Research. AHCPR Publication No. 93–0551. April 1993.
80. Rubin RR, Ciechanowski P, Egede LE, Lin EH, Lustman PJ. Recognizing and treating depression in patients with diabetes. Curr Diab Rep. 2004;4:119–25.
81. Association AD. Standards of medical care in diabetes – 2011. Diabetes Care Suppl. 2011; 1(34):S11–61.
82. Petrak F, Herpertz S, Albus C, Hirsch A, Kulzer B, Kruse J. Psychosocial Factors and Diabetes Mellitus: Evidence-Based Treatment Guidelines. Current Diabetes Reviews 2005; 1(3):255–70.
83. Arroll B, Khin N, Kerse N. Screening for depression in primary care with two verbally asked questions: cross sectional study. BMJ. 2003;327:1144–6.
84. Roy T, Lloyd CE, Pouwer F, Holt RI, Sartorius N. Screening tools used for measuring depression among people with type 1 and type 2 diabetes: a systematic review. Diabet Med. 2012; 29:164–75.
85. Awata S, Bech P, Yoshida S, et al. Reliability and validity of the Japanese version of the World Health Organization-Five Well-Being Index in the context of detecting depression in diabetic patients. Psychiatry Clin Neurosci. 2007;61:112–9.

86. Gilbody S, Bower P, Whitty P. Costs and consequences of enhanced primary care for depression: systematic review of randomised economic evaluations. Br J Psychiatry. 2006;189: 297–308.
87. Gilbody S, Sheldon T, Wessely S. Should we screen for depression? BMJ. 2006;332:1027–30.
88. Gilbody S, House AO, Sheldon TA. Screening and case finding instruments for depression. Cochrane Database Syst Rev. 2005:CD002792.
89. Pouwer F, Tack CJ, Geelhoed-Duijvestijn PH, et al. Limited effect of screening for depression with written feedback in outpatients with diabetes mellitus: a randomised controlled trial. Diabetologia. 2011;54:741–8.
90. Simon GE, Katon WJ, Lin EH, et al. Cost-effectiveness of systematic depression treatment among people with diabetes mellitus. Arch Gen Psychiatry. 2007;64:65–72.
91. Pouwer F, Snoek FJ, Van Der Ploeg HM, Ader HJ, Heine RJ. Monitoring of psychological well-being in outpatients with diabetes: effects on mood, HbA(1c), and the patient's evaluation of the quality of diabetes care: a randomized controlled trial. Diabetes Care. 2001;24:1929–35.

Chapter 2
Disentangling Clinical Depression from Diabetes-Specific Distress: Making Sense of the Mess We've Made

Sabrina A. Esbitt, Molly L. Tanenbaum, and Jeffrey S. Gonzalez

Abstract This chapter examines conceptual and applied issues regarding the screening of depression and diabetes-specific distress in adults with diabetes. We explore the conceptualization of depression as a frequently comorbid condition of diabetes and the importance of diabetes-specific distress and subthreshold depressive symptoms in regard to the emotional, behavioral, and health outcomes of living with diabetes. Overviews of the constructs of major depressive disorder (MDD) and diabetes-specific distress and challenges to an operational approach to negative emotion in the context of chronic illness are also presented in light of the meaningful overlap between diagnostic criteria of MDD and symptoms of diabetes and distress related to the burden of living with diabetes. Assessment of both depression and diabetes-specific distress are considered, including methodological issues and the strengths and weakness of leading self-report and semi-structured interview tools. Finally, suggestions for valid and clinically meaningful assessment of depressive symptoms and diabetes-specific distress in medical settings are discussed.

Keywords Diabetes • Depression • Diabetes-specific distress • Diabetes-related distress • Depression screening • Assessment

---

S.A. Esbitt, M.A. • M.L. Tanenbaum, M.A.
Ferkauf Graduate School of Psychology, Yeshiva University, Bronx, NY, USA

J.S. Gonzalez, Ph.D. (✉)
Ferkauf Graduate School of Psychology, Yeshiva University, Bronx, NY, USA

Einstein Diabetes Research Center, Albert Einstein College of Medicine, Bronx, NY, USA
e-mail: jeffrey.gonzalez@einstein.yu.edu

C.E. Lloyd et al. (eds.), *Screening for Depression and Other Psychological Problems in Diabetes*,
DOI 10.1007/978-0-85729-751-8_2, © Springer-Verlag London 2013

Introduction

Depression is increasingly recognized as a major psychosocial problem in people with diabetes. A large literature that seems to have grown exponentially over the last decade demonstrates increased prevalence of depression in diabetes patients as compared to those without diabetes [1, 2]. It also shows that depression is related to poorer diabetes self-management [3] and glycemic control [4]. While early studies showed a consistent cross-sectional relationship between depression and diabetes complications [5], leaving questions of directionality in doubt, more recent longitudinal investigations show that depression predicts the onset of complications [6–8] and mortality [6, 9, 10] over time in patients with diabetes. Based on this compelling set of findings, the importance of screening and providing treatment for depression in patients with diabetes has been emphasized, based on the reasonable expectation that identifying and treating depressed diabetes patients may result in improved diabetes outcomes. Investigations focusing on screening and treating depression in diabetes have been numerous. However, despite the rapid growth of research in this area, basic questions regarding the conceptualization and measurement of depression in diabetes continue to be the subject of considerable debate. Resolving these questions has important implications for screening and treating depression in people with diabetes.

One important question relates to the appropriateness of conceptualizing depression in diabetes as a comorbid mental illness. In the vast majority of studies that have examined depression in diabetes, the construct under investigation is major depressive disorder (MDD). Despite the consistency in application of the comorbid mental illness model to the problem of depression in diabetes, the screening measures most often used to evaluate MDD are often inadequate, have a high number of "false-positives," and may inaccurately pathologize subclinical psychological distress. We begin this chapter by providing an overview of the conceptual definition of MDD, as currently defined in the leading psychiatric diagnostic systems. We then challenge the dominance of this conceptualization and argue that the comorbidity model for MDD and diabetes mellitus has important limitations for assessment and treatment. First, we note that the current diagnostic guidelines for MDD ignore life context that may be causally related to depressive symptoms. Second, we review data showing an incremental association between depressive symptoms and diabetes outcomes, suggesting that depressive symptoms (even at subclinical levels) may be more closely associated with diabetes outcomes than MDD, per se. We also consider important findings that suggest that these symptoms are often closely related to, and in some cases predicted by, the experience of living with diabetes. Finally, we consider accumulating evidence that suggests that antidepressant therapy is ineffective for mild cases of MDD and subclinical presentations of distress.

An additional important question relates to the extent to which distress related to the burden (physical, emotional, and social) of living with diabetes may be confounded with the measurement of depression in diabetes. We describe the construct of diabetes-specific distress (DD) and discuss the problematic overlap between DD and MDD. We will make several arguments based on the available empirical literature: First, at the conceptual level, we posit that distress secondary to the burden of living with diabetes is qualitatively different from MDD, much more common

Table 2.1 Diagnostic criteria for major depression across the DSM-IV TR and the ICD-10

I.	Depressed mood
II.	Loss of interest or pleasure
III.	Fatigue or loss of energy
IV.	Decrease or increase in appetite or significant weight loss or weight gain
V.	Insomnia or hypersomnia
VI.	Psychomotor agitation or retardation
VII.	Poor concentration or indecisiveness
VIII.	Suicidal thoughts or acts
IX.	Loss of self-confidence or self-esteem
X.	Guilt or self-blame

Note: The DSM-IV TR requires the presence of at least one of the first two symptoms, as well as additional symptoms to total five or more (loss of self-confidence or self-esteem is not a symptom in the DSM-IV TR). The ICD-10 requires at least two of the first three symptoms, with the severity of the current episode indicated by the number of total symptoms (four for mild, six for moderate, and eight for severe).

among patients, and appears to be more closely related to diabetes self-management and glycemic control. Second, the screening measures typically used to evaluate MDD in the diabetes literature may often provide case-finding results that are more indicative of diabetes-specific distress than MDD. Finally, we will consider the implications of these issues for screening and treatment approaches to depression and distress in patients living with diabetes.

Major Depressive Disorder

Major depressive disorder (MDD) is the most commonly diagnosed psychiatric mood disorder in the general population [11, 12]. MDD in the Diagnostic and Statistical Manual of Mental Disorders, Fourth Edition, Text Revision (DSM-IV) and recurrent depressive disorder in the International Statistical Classification of Diseases and Related Health Problems, 10th Revision (ICD-10) reflect one or more major depressive episodes, defined by the presence of depressed mood, loss of interest, fatigue or low energy, sleep disturbance, marked increase or decrease in appetite or weight, feelings of guilt or worthlessness (in the ICD-10 also loss of confidence or self-esteem), poor concentration, psychomotor retardation or agitation, and thoughts of death or suicidality (see Table 2.1) [13, 14]. These symptoms must be present nearly every day for at least a 2-week period, and both the DSM-IV and the ICD-10 specify that they must not be due to the direct effects of a substance and a medical condition and there must be no prior experience of a manic episode. The DSM-IV additionally specifies that the symptoms must interfere with important aspects of functioning and/or cause significant distress and must not be better accounted for by bereavement [13]. The DSM-IV does recognize the possibility that presentations of major depressive episode could be due to a medical condition and offers the diagnosis of mood disorder due to a general medical condition to account for these. However, the criteria for this diagnosis are quite restrictive. For example, there must be evidence "from the history, physical examination, or laboratory findings that the disturbance is the direct physiological consequence of a general medical condition" ([13], p. 404). The requirement for a direct physiological mechanism is important, and the DSM-IV explicitly states that when the criteria for a depressive episode are met and these symptoms "are precipitated by the general medical condition acting as a psychosocial stressor, rather than resulting from the direct physiological effects of the general medical condition, the diagnosis would be Major Depressive Disorder" ([13], p. 184). Additionally, diabetes is not listed among the examples of associated general medical conditions in the DSM-IV. Thus, this diagnostic option is unlikely to be considered by most clinicians for depression in patients with diabetes.

The Role of Life Context in MDD

The DSM utilizes an operational approach to conceptualizing psychopathology, that is, an observational, rule-based approach to the identification and classification of psychiatric illness that predicates diagnosis on the presence or absence of specific symptoms [13]. The DSM-IV specifies that most life events (e.g., loss-related events other than bereavement) should not be factored into judgments of pathology when diagnosing MDD. This stands in contrast to a long history of thought from Hippocrates through to twentieth-century leaders of psychiatric theory and classification, who consistently regarded the distinction between normal loss-related sadness and pathological depression, or *melancholia*, as depending on a consideration of causal context and the proportional relation of symptom severity to this context [15]. For example, Freud acknowledged that the symptoms of bereavement and *melancholia* could be indistinguishable but emphasized the context of loss in understanding the distinction between the two experiences. As cited by Horowitz and Wakefield, he noted that "although grief involves grave departures from the normal attitude to life, it never occurs to us to regard it as a morbid condition" [16]. Similarly, and also cited by Horowitz and Wakefield, Kraepelin posited that "morbid emotions are distinguished from healthy emotions chiefly through the lack of a sufficient cause, as well as by their intensity and persistence…" [17]. Up through the DSM-II [18], which defined "depressive neurosis" as "manifested by an excessive reaction of depression due to internal conflict or to an identifiable event such as the loss of a love object or cherished possession," the question of *a disproportional* relationship between depressive symptoms and contextual explanations was central to the diagnosis of clinical depression. However, with the publication of the DSM-III [19] in 1980, the diagnostic system was significantly overhauled. Since then, DSM diagnosis has taken a neutral stance with respect to theories of etiology and the causal role of contextual factors; the current approach is largely centered on observable symptoms, isolated from context, and is aimed at increasing the consistency of diagnoses within and between clinicians [20, 21]. This focus on symptoms has resulted in increased reliability of diagnoses (e.g., if a sufficient number of specified symptoms are present, the disorder is present). However, it has also resulted in a dramatic increase in prevalence of MDD, based at least in part on the increased reach of the diagnosis into presentations of sadness that were previously considered "normal" [15]. This shift in the diagnostic approach to clinical depression has important implications for understanding distress in patients with diabetes and currently encourages clinicians to ignore the physical, emotional, and social context of living with a burdensome chronic illness when evaluating MDD.

Empirical evidence suggests that presentations of MDD, in terms of symptoms, severity, and outcomes, that are explained by contextual factors related to loss of health, economic stability, or important relationships, are similar to those presented by individuals suffering from bereavement, the only loss-related contextual factor cited by the DSM-IV which exempts an individual from diagnosis of MDD. Wakefield and colleagues [15] suggest that if MDD symptoms in the presence of bereavement are accurately exempted from diagnosis as mental illness, symptoms in the face of other significant life events may also be considered non-pathological, although others use similar data to argue for the removal of the bereavement exemption for MDD diagnosis [22]. Recent research on judgments of the pathological nature of symptoms of distress suggests that experienced clinical psychologists often approach case material in a way that contradicts the DSM-IV's direction to ignore life context. When presented with vignettes describing unaffected, mildly distressed, or disordered behaviors following either traumatic or mildly distressing life events, clinical psychologists were significantly less likely to view symptoms as abnormal when a distressing life context was present than when no context was available to explain a patient's symptom disturbance. These findings held for MDD, for which the DSM-IV instructs clinicians to ignore life context, and posttraumatic stress disorder (PTSD), for which the DSM-IV requires a preceding traumatic event [23]. A lack of appropriate distress in response to a distressing event was also seen as disordered, reflecting the importance of a *proportionate response* to life events as part of the diagnostic rubric used by experienced clinical psychologists, across theoretical orientations.

Methodological Challenges of Assessment of MDD in People with Diabetes

The conceptual murkiness surrounding the construct of depression within diabetes, as well as the structure and psychometric weaknesses of the most common MDD assessment tools, presents challenges to research and clinical practice. At the most general level of measurement problems, physical symptoms associated with diabetes, such as fatigue, poor concentration, and appetite disruption, may be mistaken for symptoms of MDD [24]. Critically, the method of assessment may also impact on the accuracy and frequency of the diagnosis of MDD. Self-report questionnaires that assess depressive symptoms are often not strongly tied to diagnostic criteria for MDD. Yet, these are used in the majority of studies examining depression or distress in diabetes despite the fact they have been found to be more representative of more general levels of distress or well-being [25].

The self-report measures that do have acceptable psychometric properties for detecting MDD often achieve sensitivity at the cost of a high false-positive rate. The implications of this problem have been clearly demonstrated in medical populations, such as in cardiovascular disease [26].

Structured clinical interviews are considered the gold standard for assessing MDD. There are several frequently used diagnostic interview schedules that assess for DSM-IV and ICD-10 psychiatric disorders, including the Mini-International Neuropsychiatric Interview (MINI; [27]), the Composite International Diagnostic Interview (CIDI) [28], and the Structured Clinical Interview for DSM (SCID) [29]. However, the administration of structured clinical interviews requires training on the part of the interviewer and is often time consuming, posing a barrier to their widespread adoption in research and clinical assessment of MDD. Roy and colleagues [24] report that 80% of studies used self-report questionnaires, with the remaining 20% using a clinical interview based on MDD criteria, in their systematic review of diabetes research studies that utilized some type of depression measurement.

Fisher et al. [30] used both the Center for Epidemiologic Studies Depression Scale (CES-D) self-report questionnaire and a structured clinical interview, the CIDI, to assess depression in patients with type 2 diabetes. Results showed that 22% of participants reached the CES-D clinical cutoff, and 10% met diagnostic criteria based on the CIDI, resulting in a 70% false-positive rate for MDD based on the CES-D. Additionally, there was a worrisome rate of false-negatives; 34% of those with MDD did not meet the CES-D cutoff. Investigations using self-report diagnostic measures have found a point prevalence of depression 200–300% higher among people with diabetes compared to those without [1], whereas studies utilizing clinical interviews paint a more conservative picture, suggesting that the prevalence of MDD is only 40–60% more common among those with diabetes compared to those without [31]. Thus, setting aside the problems with our conceptual model for MDD in diabetes discussed in the preceding section, there is strong evidence to suggest that much of the research conducted on the relationship between diabetes and depression may be biased by measurement error in the assessment of MDD. Most of the patients we call "depressed" in our research studies would not meet the criteria for MDD and a significant minority of those who we deem "not depressed" would. This has undoubtedly resulted in imprecise measurement in research on the relationship between diabetes and depression. Equally important, it has resulted in patients being incorrectly identified as clinically depressed and offered antidepressant medication, which is not indicated for subclinical distress.

Subclinical Presentations of MDD Symptoms

Although most depression research in diabetes has focused on the construct of MDD, with the above-mentioned conceptual and measurement-error caveats, it is clear that a greater risk for poor diabetes outcomes is also seen in patients with subclinical elevations of depressive symptoms compared to those with no depression, including increased risk of mortality (e.g., [6, 32]). This suggests that the experience of depressive symptoms that would not meet the diagnostic threshold for MDD is a risk factor for negative health outcomes in patients living with diabetes. Additionally, subclinical levels of depressive symptoms have been found to be 2–3 times as prevalent as clinical depression in adults with diabetes [1, 2]. Fisher and colleagues assessed patients with type 2 diabetes three times over an 18-month follow-up and found that while 20% of patients qualified for a diagnosis of MDD over that time frame, nearly 35% reported elevated symptoms of depression on the CES-D (CES-D $\geq$ 16) [31]. This elevation in symptoms of depression has been associated with poorer diabetes self-management (higher caloric intake, increased consumption of saturated fat, and decreased physical activity) in patients with type 2 diabetes, while meeting diagnostic criteria for MDD was not associated with diabetes self-management [30]. More importantly, the same elevation has also been associated with risk for diabetes complications, functional disability, and mortality over 7 years of follow-up [6]. Moreover, there was no apparent difference between the impact of MDD or subclinical depressive symptoms in predicting increased risk of negative health outcomes. Even those with "minimal depression" (CES-D = 1–15) experienced significantly increased risk for all negative health outcomes when compared to those with no symptoms of depression (CES-D = 0) [6]. These data clearly demonstrate an incremental relationship between symptoms of depression and negative health outcomes in diabetes, a relationship observed even at subclinical levels of depression severity. They challenge the model of MDD in diabetes, which conceptualizes the problem of depression as a categorical construct that is either present or not.

The concept of an incremental relationship between depressive symptoms and poor diabetes management was also examined in a survey of 879 primary care patients with type 2 diabetes [33]. Similar to the pattern observed by Black and colleagues [6] for health outcomes, results showed that self-reported depressive symptom severity predicted poor diabetes self-management behaviors (diet, exercise, and medication taking). Even among patients who scored below the screening cutoff for MDD, depressive symptom severity was still incrementally linked to poorer self-care [33]. Taken together, these findings suggest that we may be missing important avenues for clinical intervention when we focus on depression in diabetes only within the framework of MDD. While true MDD is clearly important and should be treated in patients with diabetes, subclinical presentations are much more common and are at least equivalently related to risk for poor self-management and treatment outcomes.

Diabetes as a Context for MDD

Despite being ignored by the diagnostic criteria for MDD, relationships between the lived experience of chronic illness, including diabetes, and depression have been found repeatedly throughout the literature. Clinically significant depression (CES-D $\geq$ 16) was 2.5 times more common in patients with diabetes and additional comorbid chronic illness(es) when compared to those without comorbid illness [34]. Type 2 diabetes patients who screened positive for MDD were significantly more likely to be prescribed more medications, to have a higher BMI, and to be prescribed insulin than patients who did not meet screening criteria; a nonsignificant trend for greater number of comorbid illnesses was also found in those who screened positive for MDD [33]. The presence of impairments in physical functioning, limitations of role functioning due to poor physical health, physical pain, low vitality, and impaired social functioning in a population study of people with diabetes were each significantly associated with the presence of MDD [35]. Additionally, a survey of over 30,000 individuals found that functional disability was significantly more frequent among individuals with both diabetes and MDD than those with only one of the conditions [36]. Although the directionality of these effects is unclear from these studies, a longitudinal study of community-dwelling adults showed that while illness-related physical limitations predict changes in depressive symptoms over time, depressive symptoms do not predict similar changes in physical limitations. Additionally, part of the link between physical limitations and later increases in depression appears to be explained by the experience of pain and, to a lesser degree, by the experience of social stress [37]. A study of patients with diabetic peripheral neuropathy mapped specific pathways between disease-related factors such as neuropathy severity, neuropathy-related symptoms, impairment in daily activities, and neuropathy-related limitations in important roles and increases in depressive symptoms over time, reflecting the impact of diabetes-specific experiences on mood [38]. Finally, while epidemiological data have consistently linked MDD and physical illness, these mood-illness relationships have been found to diminish with age. When chronic illness occurs in younger adults, it is more strongly associated with MDD than if it develops in older age, where the experience of illness is normative and expected, illustrating how life context is crucial for understanding the relationship between illness and depression [39, 40]. These linkages between the experience of illness and the experience of depression provide an important context to consider in evaluating the abnormality of depressive symptoms. They also provide clues to potentially fruitful avenues of intervention that target depression by reducing the burden of illness (e.g., by improving coping and adaptation to changing roles). These illness-focused opportunities for intervention may be missed by the context neutral approach to diagnosing MDD.

Diabetes-Specific Distress

If we accept that the model of MDD for understanding the problem of depression in diabetes is lacking, then how are we to conceptualize the experience of subclinical depressive symptoms in many people living with diabetes? Can we improve our accounting of the often-close linkages between the experience of diabetes and the experience of emotional distress in patients? The construct of diabetes-specific

Table 2.2 Diabetes distress scale

DDS subscales (17 items total)	Example items
Emotional burden (5 items)	"Feeling angry, scared, and/or depressed when I think about living with diabetes"
Physician-related distress (4 items)	"Feeling that my doctor doesn't give me clear enough directions on how to manage my diabetes"
Regimen-related distress (5 items)	"Not feeling motivated to keep up my diabetes self-management"
Interpersonal distress (3 items)	"Feeling that friends or family are not supportive enough of self-care efforts (e.g., planning activities that conflict with my schedule, encouraging me to eat the "wrong" foods)"

emotional distress addresses these questions. Diabetes distress is distinct from the concept of general emotional distress and was developed to specifically assess psychosocial adjustment in diabetes [41]. Diabetes-specific distress is also conceptually distinct from MDD; it is conceptualized as emotional distress that arises from living with diabetes and seen as a common psychosocial symptom of diabetes, predicated on a variety of medical, contextual, and individual factors, not on the presence of a psychiatric condition. Diabetes-specific distress can stem from a range of areas related to living with the burden of chronic illness. These may include difficult relationships with providers, feelings of failure, inadequacy or burnout related to keeping up with one's treatment regimen, conflict with family or friends due to one's illness, or frustration, anger, or sadness over living with diabetes [42]. Importantly, the concept of diabetes-specific distress is more closely aligned with patient views about the role of emotional distress in diabetes than the MDD comorbidity model. For example, results of a recent meta-synthesis of 22 qualitative studies addressing the co-occurrence of diabetes and depression found that patients associated diabetes with a variety of emotional reactions, including anger, shame, fear, shock, and guilt. Findings suggested that these emotional processes might more accurately be called diabetes-specific distress or diabetes-related demoralization than clinical depression [43].

Diabetes-specific distress – most commonly measured using the Problem Areas in Diabetes (PAID) [41] scale and the later Diabetes Distress Scale (DDS) (Tables 2.2 and 2.3) [42] – was uniquely associated with diabetes-specific outcomes and was an independent predictor of poorer diabetes self-care behavior [41]. When both structured clinical interviews for MDD and self-report questionnaires that measure diabetes-specific distress have been used, findings indicate that these measures tap into different constructs with their own independent associations with diabetes; diabetes-specific distress is closely associated with diabetes self-management and glycemic control, while MDD is not [30, 44]. Fisher and colleagues [44] found that diabetes-specific distress is linked to HbA1c both cross-sectionally and longitudinally, while MDD was not. They posit that HbA1c and diabetes-specific distress are related bidirectionally, in that they both influence each other over time. Patients with

Table 2.3 Self-report measures of diabetes-specific distress; the Problem Areas in Diabetes Scale (PAID) and the Diabetes Distress Scale (DDS)

Measure	Problem areas in diabetes (20 items)	Diabetes distress scale (17 items)
Domains	Diabetes-related emotional problems (12 items)	Emotional burden (5 items)
	Treatment problems (3)	Physician-related distress (4 items)
	Food-related problems (3)	Regimen-related distress (5 items)
	Social support-related problems (2)	Interpersonal distress (3 items)

poor glycemic control may then experience distress, which could lead to sustained poor disease management. Conversely, patients experiencing significant diabetes-specific distress may be less likely to practice self-care behaviors, which could then negatively impact their HbA1c level.

While findings have consistently shown that diabetes-specific distress is more closely associated with diabetes self-management than MDD, studies that have investigated independent relationships between diabetes distress and depressive symptoms on the one hand and diabetes self-management on the other have provided a somewhat different picture. In a cross-sectional evaluation of a large primary care sample of people with type 2 diabetes, a continuous measure of depressive symptom severity was more closely associated with poorer diabetes self-management than the PAID in multivariate models. This remained true even when those who screened positive for MDD were removed from the analysis [45]. Similarly, Lloyd and colleagues showed that CES-D score was a better independent predictor of physical activity than PAID scores in patients with type 1 diabetes [46]. Although these results may appear to contradict the idea that diabetes-specific distress accounts for the relationship between depression and diabetes self-management, caution should be used in drawing conclusions about the relative importance of the constructs of depression and diabetes-specific distress from these findings. There is substantial overlap in the measures of these constructs. For example, scores on a DSM-IV-based screener for MDD and PAID scores shared 29% of their variance in the study by Gonzalez and colleagues [45]. CES-D scores and PAID scores share 24% of their variance, and CES-D scores and DDS total scores share approximately 23% of their variance [30, 46]. This shared variance may be equally important as the unique variance in each measure but is eliminated from multiple regression analyses. More importantly, although researchers may conceptualize measures of depression as distinct from measures of diabetes-specific distress, respondents are unlikely to make such a distinction. There is no reason to believe that high scores on depression symptom measures, which contain items that reflect a more severe level of emotional distress and functional impairment than those on the PAID or DDS, could not represent distress that is caused by diabetes (as discussed above). Thus, disentangling these constructs is exceedingly difficult.

A recent study clearly demonstrates how the context of diabetes can have a causal influence on ratings of depression severity. A qualitative analysis of transcripts of structured clinical interviews for depression symptom severity, administered by a trained clinician to 34 adults with type 1 diabetes, revealed that nearly three-fourths of participants who reported symptoms of depression discussed these symptoms within a diabetes-specific context, which was indicative of either diabetes-specific distress or depressive-like symptoms (e.g., appetite, sleep, or concentration disturbances) more likely due to diabetes and effects of high or low blood sugars [47]. The diabetes-specific distress content expressed by participants during the interview fell into areas related to negative emotional reactions (e.g., anger, frustration, anxiety, depression) to high glucometer readings, feeling overwhelmed by diabetes, being upset about weight gain thought to be associated with insulin use, and guilt over burdening others with one's illness. Thus, even the gold standard of depression assessment, a structured clinical interview administered by a trained professional, may be vulnerable to influence by diabetes-specific distress. It is unknown how diabetes distress influences likelihood of misdiagnosing distress as a psychiatric disorder, but findings from this study point to the strong possibility that the presence of diabetes-specific distress complicates the assessment of MDD. Not attending to diabetes as a context, and distress that arises specifically from living with diabetes during depression assessment, could lead to an overdiagnosis of MDD or missing the presence of distress that is secondary to living with the burden of a chronic illness. These errors have implications for the selection of appropriate treatments. Before we turn to these implications, we first briefly review psychometric properties of diabetes distress measures.

Screening for Diabetes-Specific Distress

Several measures have been created to assess different aspects of diabetes-specific distress. In addition to the PAID and the DDS, these include the 39-item ATT39, which measures emotional adjustment in patients with diabetes [48], and the 45-item Questionnaire on Stress in Patients with Diabetes-Revised (QSD-R, [49]), which contains subscales that assess different potential stressful areas of living with diabetes, including leisure time, depression/fear of future, hypoglycemia, treatment regimen/diet, physical complaints, work, partner, and doctor-patient relationship [50]. In addition, the diabetes version of the Illness Perceptions Questionnaire, a self-report measure based on Leventhal's self-regulatory model of health beliefs assessing perception of illness across the domains of identity, causality, timeline, consequences, and curability/controllability, has a subscale for emotional representations of diabetes [51].

The Problem Areas in Diabetes (PAID) scale and the more recent Diabetes Distress Scale (DDS) are the most widely used measures of diabetes-specific distress [41, 42]. The PAID is a 20-item self-report instrument developed to measure diabetes-specific emotional distress across areas ranging from emotional and interpersonal distress to struggles with the diabetes management regimen [41]. It uses a 5-point Likert scale format to assess the degree to which diabetes management and/or feelings about diabetes are problematic to patients, with responses ranging from "not a problem" to a "serious problem." Initially developed in English at the Joslin Diabetes Center, Boston, USA, from data collected from diabetes health care providers and patients with diabetes, it has been translated into Spanish, Japanese,

Dutch, German, Chinese, Croatian, Danish, and Portuguese [52–54]. It was developed to aid health care providers in collaborating with patients and is primarily used to assess distress and monitor patient change. A cutoff score of 40 has been recommended to denote elevated levels of distress, with a score of 50 denoting seriously elevated distress [46, 55, 56].

While the PAID was originally developed without subscales, Snoek and colleagues [54] found that a four-factor model comprised of subscales representing diabetes-related emotional problems (12 items), treatment problems (3 items), food-related problems (3 items), and social support-related problems (2 items) presented the best fit for data from a sample of 1,696 participants from the Netherlands and the USA [54]. However, this four-factor structure has not held up in several attempts to validate international versions of the PAID, such as the Chinese [57] and Norwegian [58] versions. Additionally, a two-factor structure was found in the Turkish [59] version of the PAID (a 5-item "support-related issues" factor and a 15-item "diabetes-distress" factor), and a 7-item "lack of confidence" subscale and a 13-item "negative emotional consequences" subscale were uncovered in an investigation of the psychometric properties of the PAID among rural, African-American women [60]. Cultural variability has been suggested as a likely explanation for this variation, and an important consideration overall in the assessment of diabetes-specific distress [58, 60].

The PAID has been found to have consistently high internal reliability, good item-to-total correlations, sound 2-month test–retest reliability, and to correlate strongly with constructs it would be expected to be associated with, such as emotional distress, depression, disordered eating, fear of hypoglycemia, HbA1C, diabetes complications, and activities of diabetes self-care [41, 61]. It has not been associated with length of diabetes, education, or ethnicity, although it is negatively associated with age [41, 62, 63]. Findings regarding the relationship between diabetes-specific distress and gender have been mixed [54]. In a survey of 815 primary care patients with type 2 diabetes, patients treated with insulin evidenced higher diabetes distress on the PAID as compared with patients on a diet or oral medication treatment regimen [64]. McGuire and colleagues [65] identified two psychometrically robust short-form measures of diabetes-specific emotional distress: a reliable and brief 5-item version of the PAID (PAID-5) with good sensitivity (94%) and specificity (89%) for the recognition of diabetes-specific emotional distress and a single-item screening question ("worrying about the future and the possibility of serious complications"), the PAID-1, possessing concurrent sensitivity and specificity of 80%.

In a comparison of different measures of depression assessment among diabetes patients, including self-report measures, a structured clinical interview, a nonstructured clinical interview including psychiatric history, and a measure of diabetes-specific distress, the PAID showed superior ability to detect both clinical and subclinical depression, as well as diabetes-related distress when compared to standard measures of assessment for depression alone [55]. Higher scores on certain PAID items that reflect feelings of burnout from diabetes management and feeling depressed about diabetes were more strongly related to clinical depression, reflecting the need for targeted assessment of depression as well as diabetes-specific distress. Shortcomings of the PAID include its length and the criticism that it does not fully address diabetes distress related to patients' attitudes toward their diabetes care providers [42].

Due to these limitations of the PAID, Polonsky et al. [42] created the Diabetes Distress Scale (DDS), a 17-item measure of diabetes-specific distress that contains four subscales: emotional burden, physician-related distress, regimen-related distress, and interpersonal distress. Like the PAID, the DDS was developed with provider and patient feedback in mind; unlike the PAID, the four subscales were chosen a priori, reflecting a core conceptual stance regarding key domains of diabetes-specific distress [42]. The DDS-17 provides a total score plus 4 subscale scores. A mean score of 3 or higher has been considered moderate distress and has been used to discriminate low-distress groups from those worthy of clinical attention. Fisher and colleagues later determined more specific cutoff categories, with a mean score under 2 indicating "little or no" diabetes distress, a mean score between 2 and 2.9 indicating "moderate" diabetes distress, and a score of 3 or higher indicating "high" diabetes distress [66]. This study found increases in diabetes distress as measured by the DDS-17 to be associated with higher HbA1c, lower self-efficacy, less physical activity, and poorer diet [66].

A brief review of its psychometric properties reveals a consistent, generalizable factor structure and adequate internal reliability and validity across the four subscales ($\alpha > 0.87$) [42]. It is suggested that health care providers review the DDS-17 with the patient regardless of scores as part of a comprehensive diabetes assessment [42]. A brief 2-item diabetes distress screen based on the DDS-17 was developed by Fisher and colleagues [67], and the DDS-2 was found to have similar cutoff scores as the DDS-17 [66]. The DDS-2 is comprised of the items "feeling overwhelmed by the demands of living with diabetes" and "feeling that I am often failing with my diabetes regimen," which respondents rate on a 6-point scale. It displayed high levels of sensitivity and specificity, .95 and .85, respectively, with an accuracy rate (true positive) of 96.7% when measured against the benchmark of the DDS-17 [67]. Despite the brevity of the DDS-2, a recent examination by Fisher and colleagues of its psychometric properties found that it classified participants into categories of diabetes-specific distress similarly to the full DDS-17; a score <2 indicated little or no distress, moderate diabetes distress fell between 2 and 2.9, and ≥3 indicated high levels of diabetes distress [66]. As even relatively low levels of distress have been associated with poorer diabetes outcomes, a DDS-2 of >2 (average of the 2 items) may warrant further investigation of the patient's diabetes-specific distress, including more comprehensive assessment via administration of the DDS-17.

Where Do We Go from Here? Clinical Implications for Screening in Medical and Mental Health Settings

The importance of assessing emotional well-being and quality of life as part of the medical management of diabetes is reflected in statements from the American Diabetes Association (ADA) and International Diabetes Federation (IDF) [68, 69].

The ADA recommends that psychosocial screening take place both at sentinel moments in diabetes care, such as at diagnosis, discovery of complications, hospitalization, or problems in control or self-management, as well as part of regular follow-up. The current challenges of accurately assessing diabetes-specific distress, clinically significant depressive symptoms, and MDD should not deter us from improving how we assess and address the common experience of emotional distress in individuals living with diabetes as a component of comprehensive diabetes care. Without adequate assessment, identifying patients with depressive symptoms or diabetes-specific distress may not be clear, even among highly trained health care professionals. For example, in a study by Pouwer and colleagues [70], diabetes nurse specialists failed to recognize depression and diabetes-specific emotional distress in three-fourths of patients with high scores on the Hospital Anxiety and Depression Scale (HADS) or PAID scale. This finding demonstrates a disconnect between distress and depressive symptoms disclosed by diabetes patients via self-report compared to how they may present in the time-limited, medically oriented setting of a medical visit.

Distinguishing between MDD and diabetes distress in patients with diabetes is a necessary step to ensure appropriate treatment referrals and decisions following an elevated score on one of the several self-report tools used to identify distressed patients in clinical settings. The use of a screening methodology that results in a high rate of false-positives for MDD among patients with diabetes presents challenges to treatment planning and intervention. Roy et al. [24] point out that self-report tools should be used only as a first step to screen for symptoms that could then lead to a clinical interview. Misidentifying distressed patients with diabetes as having MDD could lead to prescribing antidepressants, which may not lead to improvement in symptoms, since they do not appear to be more effective than placebo for mild or subclinical presentations of MDD [71]. Certainly, additional targeted differential diagnosis by a trained mental health provider would be needed to confirm or disconfirm an MDD diagnosis [72]. In the current health care system, MDD and other psychiatric disorders are often treated outside of the medical context by mental health specialists who may not be well versed in the complexities of life with diabetes. This has obvious disadvantages for treatment if we accept that distress and diabetes are often causally and bidirectionally linked.

Diabetes-specific distress and subclinical depressive symptoms should be evaluated in light of the context presented by their experience with diabetes and should be screened for as part of comprehensive diabetes care. More appropriate treatment for patients with diabetes-specific distress could be targeted toward assisting patients in better managing their treatment regimen, providing peer support from others with diabetes, and additional education/guidance or encouragement in order to optimize their care and integrate mental health into disease management.

Treating the significant numbers of distressed diabetes patients within the diabetes care environment (as opposed to referring them out to separate mental health services) allows providers to have maximal impact on their patient's well-being through comprehensive, psychosocially sophisticated care [73]. Despite the importance of screening for diabetes-specific distress, the majority of literature portrays the use of the PAID and the DDS as part of the collection of descriptive or outcome data in research studies as opposed to practical tools integrated in clinical settings [44, 74]. Although there is a dearth of translational research on how to best utilize these screening tools in the practice arena, we offer some suggestions based on the diabetes-specific distress and integrative primary care literature.

For screening of diabetes-specific distress to be useful to patients and providers, it should fit into the flow of the visit and not significantly increase provider burden [75]. How to incorporate self-report measures into a time-limited visit is an important consideration. Screening is of little use if providers do not know how to use screening results in a way that improves the efficacy of the care they provide. Furthermore, medical providers may be wary of assessing affectively laden issues such as the burden of living with diabetes for fear that it will lead them into complex emotional or behavioral areas that cannot be addressed within the limits of their visit. However, talking openly about the distress related to the challenge of diabetes does not require special mental health training; empathic listening, engagement in thoughtful and supportive dialogue, and the use of reflective comments are important skills for all members of the health care team [73]. Understanding emotional distress within the context of the patient's experience of managing their diabetes supports interventions that target challenges in diabetes self-regulation, including maladaptive beliefs about diabetes or avoidance of diabetes-specific behaviors such as self-care due to illness-specific emotional distress. Incorporating emotional and behavioral management into diabetes care may be more effective and better received than approaches that focus solely on decreasing emotional symptoms without acknowledging the diabetes-relevant issues that underlie mood symptoms or the widespread approach of providing diabetes education without acknowledging the psychosocial factors that impact on the understanding and incorporation of medical information [76].

If a comprehensive approach to diabetes is to be feasible, health care providers must also have access to appropriate referrals, resources, and education; if assessment of depression or diabetes-specific distress is to occur as part of normal diabetes care, providers must feel confident that they know what to do with positive screens for MDD or diabetes-specific distress. Glasgow and colleagues [75, 77] discuss methods for translating behavior change research into primary care practice and suggest utilizing the 5 A's Behavior Change Model (Assess, Advise, Agree, Assist, and Arrange) when integrating behavioral health interventions into practice and emphasize the interdependence of these steps on each other. In the case of screening for diabetes-specific distress, assessment should be effectively integrated into the visit to maximize the value of the screen (Assess). The provider can use feedback from the assessment to target appropriate interventions based on the specific nature of the patient's distress (Advise). The patient and provider can then collaborate to set specific, measurable diabetes-specific goals and assist them in deciding on a course of action (Agree). They can assist patients by helping them to implement their goals through planning and problem-solving strategies (Assist), provide appropriate referrals, and can help arrange supports for the patient via follow-up care, following up with referrals, and ongoing assessment and intervention

(Arrange). More specific suggestions for integrating empirically validated assessment into primary care include using all the resources of a primary care practice to provide comprehensive patient care, including utilizing waiting room time for completing brief self-report assessments [75, 77]. Making data on diabetes-specific distress available prior to the start of encounters in the same manner as BMI or blood pressure readings may allow the provider a quick snapshot of their patients' adjustment to their illness allowing them to provide feedback on the patients' responses and incorporate a discussion about problem areas into the flow of the visit.

To our knowledge, no data exists that supports the use of brief self-report measures of diabetes-specific distress over an ongoing clinical conversation in which the provider addresses the patient's emotional, social, medical, and functional experience of diabetes and how they influence their self-management. By openly discussing nonpsychiatric distress in the context of diabetes, such a conversation can build trust and collaboration between the patient and provider and avoid the false-positives or pathologizing of common emotional symptoms that may result from the use of screeners geared toward detecting MDD. Conversations between patients and providers about distress may facilitate the introduction of brief interventions, such as identifying realistic goals or collaborating in problem-solving. They can also serve as opportunities for continued evaluation of the possible presence of more severe psychiatric conditions, such as MDD. Having their emotional experience of dealing with diabetes normalized by their physician or nurse can be therapeutic and foster patient engagement with their diabetes care [72]. As levels of distress may vary over time, evaluating diabetes distress should be an ongoing process with follow-up across visits, and easy access to this information in patient records increases the likelihood that these symptoms will continue to be addressed over time.

Summary

It is suggested that the modern diagnostic system for MDD, with its operational approach to assessment, overlooks the life context in which symptoms occur and leads to the overapplication of the MDD comorbidity model to the problem of distress in diabetes. While this approach may improve the reliability of diagnosis, it sacrifices ecological validity and can be particularly problematic in treating patients with diabetes, as the co-occurrence of diabetes-specific distress or subclinical depressive symptoms have been related to diabetes self-management above and beyond the presence of MDD. Individuals with diabetes presenting with depressive mood symptoms or distress specifically related to their lived experience with diabetes may be misclassified as having MDD, especially when self-report measures are used. MDD may be overdiagnosed among patients with diabetes at the expense of accurately capturing patients' experience of diabetes-specific distress. Further study dedicated to disentangling the relationship between distress specific to the burden of chronic illness and the clinical implication of comorbid MDD and diabetes is necessary, as is more rigorous and targeted use of structured clinical interviews and well-selected screening tools. In light of their relationship to diabetes self-care and health outcomes and greater prevalence than MDD, we suggest that health professionals (and patients) may be better served by assessing for distress and depressive symptoms overall and for MDD. Much work has yet to be done in developing best practices for assessing diabetes distress and developing appropriate treatment and follow-up plans within the context of an often overburdened health care system. The prevalence of distress and depressive symptoms among adults living with diabetes and the impact on self-care and medical outcomes present both a challenge and opportunity for collaborative, comprehensive, and integrative care of diabetes.

References

1. Anderson R, Freedland K, Clouse R, Lustman P. The prevalence of comorbid depression in adults with diabetes: a meta-analysis. Diabetes Care. 2001;24:1069–78.
2. Ali S, Stone MA, Peters JL, Davies MJ, Khunti K. The prevalence of co-morbid depression in adults with type 2 diabetes: a systematic review and meta-analysis. Diabet Med. 2006;23(11): 1165–73.
3. Gonzalez J, Peyrot M, McCarl L, Collins E, Serpa L, Mimiaga M, Safren S. Depression and diabetes treatment nonadherence: a meta-analysis. Diabetes Care. 2008;31:2398–403.
4. Lustman PJ, Griffith LS, Freedland KE, Clouse RE. Fluoxetine for depression in diabetes. Diabetes Care. 2000;23:618–23.
5. de Groot M, Anderson R, Freedland K, Clouse R, Lustman P. Association of depression and diabetes complications: a meta-analysis. Psychosom Med. 2001;63:619–30.
6. Black S, Markides K, Ray L. Depression predicts increased incidence of adverse health outcomes in older Mexican Americans with type 2 diabetes. Diabetes Care. 2003;26:2822–8.
7. Lin EHB, Rutter CM, Katon W, Heckbert SR, Ciechanowski P, Oliver MM, et al. Depression and advanced complications of diabetes: a prospective cohort study. Diabetes Care. 2010;33: 264–9.
8. Gonzalez JS, Esbitt SA. Depression and treatment nonadherence in type 2 diabetes: assessment issues and an integrative treatment approach. Epidemiol Psichiatr Soc. 2010;19(2): 110–5.
9. Egede L. Effect of depression on self-management behaviors and health outcomes in adults with type 2 diabetes. Curr Diabetes Rev. 2005;1(3):235–43.
10. Katon WJ, Fan MY, Unützer J, Taylor J, Pincus H, Schoenbaum M. Depression and diabetes: a potentially lethal combination. J Gen Intern Med. 2008;23:1571–5.
11. Katon WJ, Ciechanowski P. The impact of major depression on chronic medical illness. J Psychosom Res. 2002;53:859–63.
12. Moscicki EK. Epidemiology of completed and attempted suicide: towards a framework for prevention. Clin Neurosci Res. 2001;1:310–23.
13. American Psychiatric Association. Diagnostic and statistical manual of mental disorders. 4th ed. Washington, DC: American Psychiatric Association; 2000.
14. World Health Organization. ICD-10 classifications of mental and behavioural disorder: clinical descriptions and diagnostic guidelines. Geneva: World Health Organization; 2010.
15. Horowitz AV, Wakefield JC. The loss of sadness: how psychiatry transformed normal sorrow into depressive disorder. New York: Oxford University Press; 2007.
16. Freud S. Mourning and melancholia. In: Strachey J, editor. The standard edition of the complete works of Sigmund Freud, vol. 14. London: Hogarth Press; 1917/1957. p. 152–70.
17. Diefendorf AR, Kraepelin E. Clinical psychiatry: abstracted and adapted from the seventh German edition of Kraepelin's "Lehrbuch der Psychiatrie". New York: Macmillan; 1907/1915.

18. American Psychiatric Association. Diagnostic and statistical manual of mental disorders. 2nd ed. Washington, DC: American Psychological Association; 1968.
19. American Psychiatric Association. Diagnostic and statistical manual of mental disorders. 3rd ed. Washington, DC: American Psychological Association; 1980.
20. American Psychiatric Association. Diagnostic and statistical manual of mental disorders. 4th ed. Washington, DC: American Psychological Association; 1994.
21. Kihlstrom JF. To honor Kraepelin: from symptoms to pathology in the diagnosis of mental illness. In: Beutler LE, Malik ML, editors. Rethinking the DSM: a psychological perspective. Washington, DC: American Psychological Association; 2002.
22. Kendler K, Myers J, Zisook S. Does bereavement-related major depression differ from major depression associated with other stressful life events? Am J Psychiatry. 2008;165:1449–55.
23. Kim NS, Paulus DJ, Gonzalez JS, Khalife D. Proportionate responses to life events influence clinicians' judgments of psychological abnormality. Psychol Assess. doi:10.1037/a0026416.
24. Roy T, Lloyd CE, Pouwer F, Holt RIG, Sartorius N. Screening tools used for measuring depression among people with type 1 and type 2 diabetes: a systematic review. Diabet Med. 2012; 29(2):164–75.
25. Coyne JC. Self-reported distress: analog or ersatz depression? Psychol Bull. 1994;116:29–45.
26. Thombs BD, de Jonge P, Coyne JC, Whooley MA, Frasure-Smith N, Mitchell AJ, et al. Depression screening and patient outcomes in cardiovascular care: a systematic review. JAMA. 2008;300:2161–71.
27. Sheehan DV, Lecrubier Y, Sheehan KH, et al. The mini-international neuropsychiatric interview (M.I.N.I.): the development and validation of a structured diagnostic psychiatric interview for DSM-IV and ICD-10. J Clin Psychiatry. 1998;59(20):22–33.
28. Wittchen HU. Reliability and validity studies of the WHO–composite international diagnostic interview (CIDI): a critical review. J Psychiatr Res. 1994;28(1):57–84.
29. First MB, Frances A, Pincxus HA. DSM-IV handbook of differential diagnosis. Washington, DC: American Psychiatric Press; 1995.
30. Fisher L, Skaff M, Mullan J, Arean P, Mohr D, Masharani U, et al. Clinical depression versus distress among patients with type 2 diabetes: not just a question of semantics. Diabetes Care. 2007;30:542–8.
31. Fisher L, Skaff M, Mullan J, Arean P, Glasgow R, Masharani U. A longitudinal study of affective and anxiety disorders, depressive affect and diabetes distress in adults with type 2 diabetes. Diabet Med. 2008;25:1096–101.
32. Katon WJ, Rutter C, Simon G, Lin E, Ludman E, Ciechanowski P, et al. The association of comorbid depression with mortality in patients with type 2 diabetes. Diabetes Care. 2005;28(11): 2668–72.
33. Gonzalez J, Safren S, Cagliero E, Wexler D, Delahanty L, Wittenberg E, Blais M, Meigs J, Grant R. Depression, self-care, and medication adherence in type 2 diabetes: relationships across the full range of symptom severity. Diabetes Care. 2007;30:2222–7.
34. Pouwer F, Beekman ATF, Nijpels G, et al. Rates and risks for co-morbid depression in patients with type 2 diabetes mellitus: results of a community-based study. Diabetologia. 2003;46: 892–8.
35. Goldney RD, Phillips PJ, Fisher LJ, Wilson DH. Diabetes, depression, and quality of life: a population study. Diabetes Care. 2004;27(5):1066–70.
36. Egede L. Effects of depression on work loss and disability bed days in individuals with diabetes. Diabetes Care. 2004;27:1751–3.
37. Gayman MD, Turner RJ, Cui M. Physical limitations and depressive symptoms: exploring the nature of the association. J Gerontol B Psychol Sci Soc Sci. 2008;63:S219–28.
38. Vileikyte L, Peyrot M, Gonzalez J, Rubin R, Garrow A, Stickings D, et al. Predictors of depressive symptoms in persons with diabetic peripheral neuropathy: a longitudinal study. Diabetologia. 2009;52:1265–73.
39. Kessler RC, Birnbaum H, Bromet E, Hwang I, Sampson N, Shahly V. Age differences in major depression: results from the national comorbidity survey replication (NCS-R). Psychol Med. 2010;40:225–37.

40. Schnittker J. Chronic illness and depressive symptoms in late life. Soc Sci Med. 2005;60:13–23.
41. Polonsky WH, Anderson BJ, Lohrer PA, Welch G, Jacobson AM, Aponte JE, et al. Assessment of diabetes-related distress. Diabetes Care. 1995;18:754–60.
42. Polonsky WH, Fisher L, Earles J, Dudl RJ, Lees J, Mullan J, et al. Assessing psychosocial stress in diabetes: development of the diabetes distress scale. Diabetes Care. 2005;28:626–31.
43. Gask L, Macdonald W, Bower P. What is the relationship between diabetes and depression? A qualitative meta-synthesis of patient experience of co-morbidity. Chron Illn. 2011;7:239–52.
44. Fisher L, Mullan J, Arean P, Glasgow R, Hessler D, Masharani U. Diabetes distress but not clinical depression or depressive symptoms is associated with glycemic control in both cross-sectional and longitudinal analyses. Diabetes Care. 2010;33:23–8.
45. Gonzalez J, Delahanty L, Safren S, Meigs J, Grant R. Differentiating symptoms of depression from diabetes-specific distress: relationships with self-care in type 2 diabetes. Diabetologia. 2008;51:1822–5.
46. Lloyd CE, Pambianco G, Orchard TJ. Does diabetes-related distress explain the presence of depressive symptoms and/or poor self-care in individuals with type 1 diabetes? Diabet Med. 2010;27(2):234–7.
47. Tanenbaum ML, Gonzalez JS. The influence of diabetes distress on a clinician-rated assessment of depression in adults with type 1 diabetes. (In Press).
48. Dunn SM, Smartt H, Beeney L, Turtle J. Measurement of emotional adjustment in diabetic patients: validity and reliability of ATT39. Diabetes Care. 1986;9:480–9.
49. Herschbach P, Duran G, Waadt S, Zettler A, Amm C, Marten-Mittag B. Psychometric properties of the questionnaire on stress in patients with diabetes-revised (QSD-R). Health Psychol. 1997;16:171–4.
50. Duran G, Herschbach P, Waadt S, Strain F, Zettler A. Assessing daily problems with diabetes: a subject-oriented approach to compliance. Psychol Rep. 1995;76:515–21.
51. Moss-Morris R, Weinman J, Petrie KJ, Horne R, Cameron LD, Buick D. The revised illness perception questionnaire (IPQ-R). Psychiatry Health. 2002;17(1):1–16.
52. Ishii H, Welch GW, Jacobson A, Goto M, Okazaki K, Yamamoto T, Tsujii S. The Japanese version of the problem areas in diabetes scale: a clinical and research tool for the assessment of emotional functioning among diabetic patients. Diabetes. 1999;48:A319.
53. Lerman-Garber I, Barron-Uribe C, Calzada-Leon R, Mercado-Atri M, Vidal-Tarnayo R, Quintana S, Hernandez ME, Ruiz-Reyes MdlR, Tamez-Gutierrez LE, Nishimura-Meguro E, Villa AR. Emotional dysfunction associated with diabetes in Mexican adolescents and young adults with type-1 diabetes. Salud Publica Mex. 2003;45:13–8.
54. Snoek FJ, Pouwer F, Welch GW, Polonsky WH. Diabetes-related emotional distress in Dutch and U.S. diabetic patients: cross-cultural validity of the problem areas in diabetes scale. Diabetes Care. 2000;23:1305–9.
55. Hermanns N, Kulzer B, Krichbaum M, Kubiak T, Haak T. How to screen for depression and emotional problems in patients with diabetes: comparison of screening characteristics of depression questionnaires, measurement of diabetes-specific emotional problems and standard clinical assessment. Diabetologia. 2006;49:469–77.
56. van Bastelaar KMP, Pouwer F, Geelhoed-Duijvestijn PHLM, Tack CJ, Bazelmans E, Beekman AT, Heine RJ, Snoek FJ. Diabetes-specific emotional distress mediates the association between depressive symptoms and glycaemic control in type 1 and type 2 diabetes. Diabet Med. 2011;27(7):798–803.
57. Huang M, Courtney M, Edwards H, McDowell J. Validation of the Chinese version of the problem areas in diabetes (PAID-C) scale. Diabetes Care. 2010;33:38–40.
58. Graue M, Haugstvedt A, Wentzel-Larsen T, Iversen MM, Karlsen B, Rokne B. Diabetes-related emotional distress in adults: reliability and validity of the Norwegian versions of the problem areas in diabetes scale (PAID) and the diabetes distress scale (DDS). Int J Nurs Stud. 2012;49(2):174–82.
59. Huis In 'T Veld EMJ, Makine C, Nouwen A, Karsidag C, Kadioglu P, Karsidag K, Pouwer F. Validation of the Turkish version of the problem areas in diabetes scale. Cardio Psych Neurol. 2011, p. 6. Article ID 315068. doi: 10.1155/2011/315068.

60. Miller SA, Elasy TA. Psychometric evaluation of the problem areas in diabetes (PAID) survey in Southern, rural African American women with type 2 diabetes. BMC Public Health. 2008;8(70):1–6.
61. Weinger K, Jacobson AM. Psychosocial and quality of life correlates of glycemic control during intensive treatment of type 1 diabetes. Patient Educ Couns. 2001;42:123–31.
62. Welch GW, Jacobson AM, Polonsky WH. The problem areas in diabetes scale: an evaluation of its clinical utility. Diabetes Care. 1997;20:760–6.
63. Welch G, Weinger K, Anderson B, Polonsky WH. Responsiveness of the problem areas in diabetes (PAID) questionnaire. Diabet Med. 2003;20:69–72.
64. Delahanty LM, Grant RW, Wittenberg E, Bosch JL, Wexler DJ, Cagliero E, Meigs JB. Association of diabetes-related emotional distress with diabetes treatment in primary care patients with type 2 diabetes. Diabet Med. 2007;24(1):48–54.
65. McGuire B, Morrison T, Hermanns N, Skovlund S, Eldrup E, Gagliardino J, et al. Short-form measures of diabetes-related emotional distress: the problem areas in diabetes scale (PAID)-5 and PAID-1. Diabetologia. 2010;53(1):66–9.
66. Fisher L, Hessler DM, Polonsky WH, Mullan J. When is diabetes distress meaningful? Establishing cut points for the diabetes distress scale. Diabetes Care. 2012;35(2):259–64.
67. Fisher L, Glasgow R, Mullan JT, Skaff MM, Polonsky WH. Development of a brief diabetes distress screening instrument. Ann Fam Med. 2008;6(3):246–52.
68. American Diabetes Association. Standards of medical care in diabetes – 2011. Diabetes Care. 2011;34:S11–61.
69. International Diabetes Federation. Clinical guidelines task force, global guidelines for type 2 diabetes. Brussels: International Diabetes Federation; 2005.
70. Pouwer F, Beekman AT, Lubach C, Snoek FJ. Nurses' recognition and registration of depression, anxiety and diabetes-specific emotional problems in outpatients with diabetes mellitus. Patient Educ Couns. 2006;60:235–40.
71. Fournier JC, DeRubeis RJ, Hollon SD, Dimidjian S, Amsterdam JD, Shelton RC, et al. Antidepressant drug effects and depression severity: a patient-level meta-analysis. JAMA. 2010;303:47–53.
72. Bhui K, Bhugra D. Transcultural psychiatry: some social and epidemiological research issues. Int J Soc Psychiatry. 2001;47:1–9.
73. Gonzalez J, Fisher L, Polonsky W. Depression in diabetes: have we been missing something important? Diabetes Care. 2011;34(1):236–9.
74. Glasgow RE, Strycker LA. Level of preventive practices for diabetes management: patient, physician, and office correlates in two primary care samples. Am J Prev Med. 2000;19:9–14.
75. Glasgow RE, Lichtenstein E, Marcus AC. Why don't we see more translation of health promotion research to practice? Rethinking the efficacy to effectiveness transition. Am J Public Health. 2003;93:1261–7.
76. Detweiler-Bedell JB, Friedman MA, Leventhal H, Miller IW, Leventhal EA. Integrating co-morbid depression and chronic physical disease management: identifying and resolving failures in self-regulation. Clin Psychol Rev. 2008;28:1426–46.
77. Glasgow RE, Goldstein MG, Ockene J, Pronk NP. Translating what we have learned into practice: principles and hypotheses for addressing multiple behaviors in primary care. Am J Prev Med. 2004;27:88–110.

Chapter 3
Key Concepts in Screening for Depression in People with Diabetes

Richard I.G. Holt and Christina M. Van der Feltz-Cornelis

Abstract The prevalence of depression is increased in people with diabetes. This has led to calls for screening for depression in individuals with diabetes. The UK National Screening Committee has produced criteria for appraising the viability, effectiveness, and appropriateness of screening programs. Most criteria for screening of depression in diabetes are fully or partially fulfilled. As most screening is currently opportunistic and there are no formal screening programs, some criteria are not satisfied. There is a rationale to introduce screening for depression, but further research is needed to evaluate the most clinically effective and cost-effective way of doing so.

Keywords Depression • Diabetes • Criteria • Viability • Effectiveness Appropriateness • Screening programs • Clinical • Questionnaire

R.I.G. Holt, M.A., MB BChir, Ph.D., FRCP, FHEA (✉)
Human Development and Health Academic Unit, Faculty of Medicine,
University of Southampton, Southampton, Hampshire, UK
e-mail: righ@soton.ac.uk

C.M. Van der Feltz-Cornelis, M.D., Ph.D. Psychiatry, M.Sc. Epidemiology
Faculty of Social Sciences, Tilburg University,
90531, 5000 LE, Tilburg, The Netherlands

Topclinical Care Center for Body, Mind, and Health, GGz Breburg,
Tilburg, The Netherlands

Trimbos Instituut, Utrecht, The Netherlands

C.E. Lloyd et al. (eds.), *Screening for Depression and Other Psychological Problems in Diabetes*,
DOI 10.1007/978-0-85729-751-8_3, © Springer-Verlag London 2013

Introduction

It is well recognized that the prevalence of depression is increased in people with diabetes, whether assessed by self-administered questionnaire or by more rigorous diagnostic interviews [1]. Depression has been traditionally viewed as an understandable reaction to the diagnosis of a lifelong condition that places both considerable lifestyle and treatment demands on the person with diabetes and is associated with long-term complications and shortened life expectancy. This view is, however, too simplistic as recent studies have suggested that hyperglycemia may have an adverse effect on brain function [2] while microvascular damage in the brain may predispose an individual to depression as well as cognitive defects [3]. The importance of microvascular complications is also suggested by the increase in comorbid depression in those with other diabetes complications, especially neuropathy [4].

Comorbid depression not only impairs quality of life but also adversely affects diabetes outcomes, leading to poor glycemic control, more frequent microvascular and macrovascular complications and premature mortality [5]. Given the effects of depression in people with diabetes and the availability of effective treatment for this comorbidity [6], there is a case for screening for this often ignored complication of diabetes. Regular screening for depression in people with diabetes is now recommended by several professional bodies including the International Diabetes Federation [7], the American Diabetes Association [8], and the UK National Institute for Health and Clinical Excellence [9]. The aim of this chapter is to determine to what extent screening is justified by considering this with reference to the UK National Screening Committee criteria for appraising the viability, effectiveness, and appropriateness of a screening program (Table 3.1) [10]. Ideally, all criteria should be met before screening for a condition is initiated. At present, however, formal screening programs do not exist; most screening occurs opportunistically during health care consultations.

The Condition

1. The condition should be an important health problem.

Diabetes

Diabetes mellitus is a complex metabolic disorder characterized by persistent hyperglycemia resulting from defects in insulin secretion, insulin action, or both. The two main types of diabetes are type 1 (formerly known as insulin-dependent diabetes) and type 2 (formerly known as non-insulin-dependent diabetes). It is a major global

Table 3.1 The degree to which screening for depression in people with diabetes meets the UK national screening committee criteria

Criterion	
Important health problem	++
Natural history understood	++
Primary prevention implemented	++
Simple, safe, precise, and validated screening test	++
Distribution and cutoff test values agreed	++
Acceptability of test	+
Need for further diagnostic investigation agreed	++
Effective treatment	++
Who should receive treatment	++
Optimal clinical management and patient outcomes	+
Screening shown to be effective	–
Acceptability of screening program	+
Potential for harm	?
Cost-effectiveness	–
Quality assurance	–
Adequate staffing	+
Other options considered	+
Information about screening	+
Widening of screening program	?

++ Fully met, + partially met, – not met

health problem and in 2011 was estimated by the International Diabetes Federation to affect 366 million worldwide; both type 1 and type 2 diabetes are increasing, and this figure is projected to rise to 552 million by 2030 [11]. The increase is a result of changing population demographics, such as ageing and urbanization, and changes in diet and physical activity, in part mediated through an increase in the prevalence of obesity, and other lifestyle factors [12].

While diabetes is increasing on every continent, it is now recognized that low- and middle-income countries face the greatest burden of diabetes, as around two-thirds of those affected by diabetes live in these areas of the world. The highest absolute numbers of people with diabetes and the percentage of the population with diabetes are found in countries with developing or transitioning economies.

Diabetes is the fifth leading cause of death worldwide, accounting for 4.6 million deaths annually and outnumbering the global deaths from HIV/AIDS [13]. The premature mortality is predominantly driven by an increase in cardiovascular disease, but diabetes also causes considerable morbidity through its microvascular complications that affect the eye, nerve, and kidney. Microvascular complications affect over 80% of individuals with diabetes and are present in 20–50% of patients with newly diagnosed type 2 diabetes [14]. Diabetic retinopathy is the commonest cause of blindness in the working population in the Western world, while 20–44% of new patients requiring renal replacement therapy have diabetes. Neuropathy affects 20–50% of patients with type 2 diabetes and may lead to foot ulceration and amputation.

The economic and social costs of diabetes are enormous, both for health care services and through loss of productivity. In most developed countries, at least 10% of the total health budget is spent on the management of diabetes and its complications.

Depression

Depression is one of the commonest mental health problems affecting between 3% and 5% of the population at any time; women are more commonly affected than men. Almost one in five people can expect to experience a depressive disorder at some point in their lifetime. Its prevalence appears to be increasing such that the World Health Organization (WHO) has estimated that it will be the second leading cause of global disability (after heart disease) by 2020 [15]. The prevalence of depression doubled among US adults between 1992 and 2002.

Depression can be defined as major or minor depressive disorder (MDD) according to DSM-IV criteria [16]. It is characterized by two core symptoms, namely sustained lowered mood and markedly diminished interest or pleasure in all, or almost all, activities for most of the day over a period of at least 2 weeks. Furthermore, at least four other symptoms and signs should be present, encompassing both psychological symptoms and biological changes, to define major depression. The psychological symptoms include a predominance of negative thinking or cognitions, such as hopelessness, worthlessness, and unwarranted guilt within the individual. When profound, this hopelessness may extend to suicidal ruminations, plans, and attempts to end life which are not infrequently fatal. Concentration is often diminished, and the individual may report sleep disturbance, classically with early-morning awakening, loss of appetite, lowered libido, and a lack of enjoyment of usual pleasurable activities (anhedonia). Energy levels are often decreased, and the individual reports a lack of motivation for even the most routine day-to-day tasks. Minor depression is defined as a mood disorder that does not meet full criteria for major depression but in which at least two core depressive symptoms are present for 2 weeks.

Depression is associated with increased all-cause mortality across a broad range of physical diseases as well as traumatic deaths and suicide. In particular, attention has been paid to the increase in cardiovascular mortality in those with depression; depression increases the risk of cardiovascular disease by 1.5–2.0-fold in both men and women, independent of other risk factors [17], and worsens survival post-myocardial infarction when depression is associated with a 2.25-fold increased risk of all-cause mortality and 2.71-fold increased risk of cardiac mortality [18].

The economic costs of depression are considerable; in addition to the increasing costs of antidepressant treatment, it also accounts for significant long-term sickness. In 2000, an international comparison of costs in the USA and UK found that depression costs a total of US$ 65 billion in the USA at 1998 prices, while direct costs in the UK were £417 million [19]. Within the direct costs, hospitalization was the major cost, accounting for 43–75% of the average per patient cost. A more recent study undertaken by the independent research service of the UK House of Commons

Library estimated that the cost to the British economy had risen from £5.2 billion in 1999 to £8.6 billion a year in 2009 [20].

Comorbid Depression in Diabetes

Comorbid depression in diabetes occurs frequently, with a range of 10–31% [1]. In general, somatic-psychiatric comorbidity is associated with increased morbidity and mortality, largely caused by preventable or treatable medical conditions such as metabolic disorders, such as diabetes, and cardiovascular disease as well as a high prevalence of modifiable risk factors including obesity and smoking. Despite its importance, this comorbidity often remains unrecognized and undertreated, especially in the case of comorbid depression [21]. Patients with such comorbidity die on average 25 years earlier in schizophrenia and bipolar and unipolar affective disorder, even after adjustment for suicide [22].

2. **The epidemiology and natural history of the condition, including development from latent to declared disease, should be adequately understood, and there should be a detectable risk factor, disease marker, latent period, or early symptomatic stage.**

Epidemiology of Diabetes and Depression

Both diabetes and depression are common conditions, and therefore, a degree of co-occurrence would be expected purely by chance. There is overwhelming evidence, however, that depression occurs more frequently than expected in people with diabetes. Whether determined by self-report or more stringent diagnostic interview, the rates of depression are around twofold higher in people with diabetes, with as many as 30% of individuals reporting depressive symptoms [1].

Historically, the prevalence of depression in people with diabetes has been assessed numerous times, but many of the early studies had significant methodological shortcomings. As well as lack of standardized definitions of depression, studies tended to ignore the heterogeneity of people with diabetes, mixing populations of people with type 1 and type 2 diabetes. Older studies frequently selected patients from particular settings, such as hospital outpatient clinics, where the prevalence of depression might be expected to be higher than in a wider population of people with diabetes. Further bias may have been added by low or unknown response rates.

More recent studies, using better methods, and meta-analyses have led to lower but more accurate estimates of prevalence [1]. At least in type 2 diabetes, it seems that women are more likely to develop depression than men, but the consequences appear to be worse in men with diabetes. Depression is commoner in those with diabetes complications, particularly painful neuropathy, and in people receiving insulin therapy [4, 23]. Other diabetes-specific risk factors include recurrent hypoglycemia and poor glycemic control.

The incidence of depression is also higher in people with diabetes; a recent meta-analysis of 11 studies including nearly 50,000 people with type 2 diabetes but without depression at baseline found the relative risk of depression was increased by 24% [24].

Consequences of Comorbid Diabetes and Depression

Comorbid depression not only impairs quality of life but also adversely affects diabetes outcomes [5]. A postal survey of 4,168 patients with diabetes found that the 487 people with major depression ($N=487$) reported significantly more diabetes symptoms than those without depression, with the overall number of diabetes symptoms correlating with the number of depressive symptoms [25].

People with depression show poorer self-care behavior; diet and exercise advice is followed less rigorously, and patients are less likely to self-monitor their glucose or take medications as prescribed [26]. Cross-sectional studies have indicated that people with depression have poorer glycemic control [27, 28], and depression is associated with an increased number and severity of microvascular and macrovascular complications [29]. Furthermore, even if the depression is relatively mild, it is associated with shortened life expectancy [30]. Both direct and indirect health costs increase in those with comorbid depression and diabetes [31].

The Development from Latent to Declared Disease

The management of diabetes has a number of aims; first, life-threatening diabetes emergencies, such as hypoglycemia and diabetic ketoacidosis, should be managed effectively and ideally prevented. Symptoms of hyperglycemia, such as polyuria and polydipsia, should be addressed. In the longer term, effective diabetes management should reduce its complications through screening and improved glycemic control and cardiovascular risk factor management.

The pathogenesis of diabetes complications is not fully understood and is likely to be multifactorial. Prolonged exposure to hyperglycemia undoubtedly predisposes to the generation of microvascular complications, while there may be a “U” shaped relationship between mean updated hemoglobin and macrovascular events [32, 33]. Intervention studies in people with either type 1 or type 2 diabetes have shown that improved glycemic control is associated with a reduction in the incidence and progression of microvascular complications [14, 34]. Treating marked hyperglycemia also reduces the number of cardiovascular events and mortality although it takes longer for these benefits to accrue [35, 36]. Attempts to normalize glucose in those with more modest hyperglycemia, however, have been associated with either no effect or increased overall mortality [37–40]. Consequently, rigorous attention to other cardiovascular risk factors is needed to lower the risk of cardiovascular disease.

Epidemiological studies suggest that depression is associated with an increased prevalence of complications [4]. Most of these studies are cross-sectional, and so we cannot conclude with certainty that depression is a risk factor for the development of complications. One longitudinal cohort study of 66 people with type 1 diabetes, however, found that depression was an independent risk factor for retinopathy at 10 years [41], while a further study reported that patients with a lifetime history of any affective disorder had greater progression of retinopathy than patients with no psychiatric history [42]. Although the findings of these two studies support the hypothesis that depression may accelerate the development of diabetes complications, other studies have had negative results. Nevertheless, it may be expected that depression would lead to complications through poorer glycemic control, lower rates of concordance with medication prescription, and less healthy behavior.

There Should be a Detectable Risk Factor, Disease Marker, Latent Period, or Early Symptomatic Stage

In terms of the development of major depression in diabetes, behavioral signs, such as social withdrawal, and diminished diabetes self-management, such as difficulties in following the recommended diet, are clinically detectable risk factors of a latent period of depression. Illness signs, such as high symptom burden compared to other patients with similarly advanced diabetes, can be signs of a latent period during the development of depression. Several validated questionnaires exist that can identify feelings of diabetes-related distress that may be an indication of an early symptomatic stage of depression in diabetes [43].

3. **All the cost-effective primary prevention interventions should have been implemented as far as practicable.**

Although depression is generally not a preventable condition per se, lifestyle can play a part in its progression. As well as improving glycemic control, physical activity may improve depressive symptoms, and people with diabetes should be encouraged to take at least 30 min of exercise, three to five times a week [9]. Eating a healthy diet and moderating alcohol consumption may also be helpful.

Social support may help people cope with the demands of their diabetes. Those who suffer from depression tend to withdraw from friendships and relationships, causing loneliness and isolation. Maintaining networks of family and friends may prevent this from happening.

The diagnosis of diabetes may provoke a grief reaction, and support is needed from the diabetes team to help the person with diabetes through this. Engagement is needed to help the person with diabetes come to terms with their diabetes and take control rather than being left with the feeling that their diabetes or their health care team is taking control of them. Emotional and psychological support is therefore essential.

Although no research is available indicating the cost-effectiveness of the combination of these primary preventive interventions in terms of incidence of depression in people with diabetes, programs in which diabetes nurses provide monitoring and support aimed at improved self-management have been implemented widely. One such pilot in the Netherlands evaluating such a model showed its feasibility [44].

The Test

4. There should be a simple, safe, precise, and validated screening test.

Despite of the adverse effects of comorbid depression on the individual with diabetes, there is ongoing debate about the most appropriate way to identify people with depression. Identification of people with depression can be attained by the actual diagnosis by a physician in the clinical setting, by a classifying structured interview by trained personnel, by a case-finding approach in the clinical setting, or by screening procedures performed at various levels of intensity at specialist clinic, primary care, or population levels.

Diagnosing depression by the clinician requires an index of suspicion that comorbid depression might exist in the patient. Classifying a patient as depressed requires a formal validated interview method such as the Composite International Diagnostic Interview (CIDI) or the Mini International Neuropsychiatric Interview (MINI) to elicit the symptoms of depression [45, 46]. This process is time-consuming and is unsuitable for population screening or for screening of large numbers in primary care or clinic settings. Consequently, quick and cheaper methods are needed; in response to this demand, numerous brief screening instruments or questionnaires have been developed for depression that are simple to administer and have reasonable clinical specificity and sensitivity (Table 3.2) [47–49].

A recent systematic review of depression screening tools in people with diabetes [50] found that the Beck Depression Inventory [47] and the Center for Epidemiologic Studies Depression Scale [48] were the most popular screening tools used in 24% and 21% of studies, respectively. Two further depression screening tools frequently cited in the published literature were the Patient Health Questionnaire (PHQ) (11%) [49] and the Hospital Anxiety and Depression Scale (HADS) (10%) [51]. Only a small number of studies reported reliability data, most of which showed moderate-good sensitivity but a high rate of false positives.

As there is considerable overlap between the symptoms of diabetes and depression, including tiredness, lethargy, lack of energy, sleeping difficulties, and appetite changes, it is important that any tool a clinician uses can differentiate the two conditions. Among the screening tools mentioned above, only the PHQ-9 has been well validated in patients with diabetes as well as the general population [52]; however, in patients with diabetes, the cutoff for major depression may need to be increased by 2 to 12 points or more compared with the general population where

Table 3.2 Reported sensitivity, specificity, positive and negative predictive value, and reliability and validity in tools screening for depression in people with diabetes

Tool	Sensitivity (%)	Specificity (%)	PPV (%)	NPV (%)	Reliability/validity (α)
CES-D	60.0–100	86.7	28.6	97.0	0.80
CES-D					
- Chinese	98.8	67.6	34.5	99.2	–
- Malay	66.7	60.6	23.5	90.9	–
- Indian	100	64.5	56.0	100	–
PHQ-9	66.0–100	52.0–80.0	43.8–64.4	93.4–100	0.80–0.84
BDI/SF	88.0	71.0	22.0	98.0	0.89
BDI	82.0–90.0	84.0–89.0	59.0–89.0	82.0–97.0	
HADS	74.0–85.0	37.5–86.0	28.0–49.0	95.0–96.0	0.55–0.78
Zung-SDS	69.0–100	59.0–95.0	–	–	0.72–0.88
HDRS	80.0	–	–	–	–
PAID	80.0–94.0	80.0–89.0	–	–	–
WHO-5	33.0–100.0	5.0–89.0	8.0–45.5	24.0–100	0.82–0.89
GDS	93.3	92.3	–	–	0.87

Adapted from Roy et al. [50]
Sensitivity = number of true positives (cases of depression)/number of true positives + number of false negatives
Specificity = number of true negatives/number of true negatives + false positives
Positive predictive value (PPV) = the proportion of cases with positive test results who are correctly diagnosed
Negative predictive value (NPV) = the proportion of cases with negative test results who are correctly diagnosed

the cutoff is 10 points. This adjustment allows the instrument to discriminate more accurately between diabetes-related symptoms and depressive symptoms [53]. The PHQ-9 is the shortest questionnaire of the four listed above and contains nine questions that can be completed as a self-report; these features make it easy to administer in clinics and primary care as well as population settings.

An alternative, easy, and simple method that can be used in a diabetes clinic is to ask two simple questions that explore if the patient suffers from the core symptoms of major depression [54]:

- "During the past month, have you been bothered by having little interest or pleasure in doing things?"
- "During the past month, have you been bothered by feeling down, depressed, or hopeless?"

If the answer to either is "yes," the patient should be asked if they want help with this problem. If the answer to this is also "yes," then the patient should be formally assessed by a diagnostic interview and offered appropriate treatment.

5. The distribution of test values in the target population should be known and a suitable cutoff level defined and agreed.

Each of the screening tools has cutoff values above which the risk of depression increases [47–49, 51, 53]. These have been widely published and validated in the general population. People with elevated scores should be referred promptly for a clinical diagnostic interview.

6. The test should be acceptable to the population.

While the tests are easy to administer and people with diabetes seem willing to undertake the questionnaires, it is unclear whether the indiscriminate use of the tests will lead to improved diabetes and depression outcomes.

In a randomized controlled trial investigating the benefits of depression screening in people with diabetes in the Netherlands, written feedback was provided to both patient and doctor following screening by the CIDI [55]. The intervention had little effect on the use of mental health services and did not improve depression scores compared with routine care. A further study found that screening per se was insufficient to change the recognition and treatment behavior of the physician [56].

This suggests that simply providing information after screening is insufficient to improve clinical outcomes, and more intensive depression management is required; however, this may not be acceptable to patients as in a validation study and randomized clinical trial performed in diabetes clinics, many patients identified with depression by screening did not want to undertake more intensive treatment for their comorbid depression [53].

Consequently, screening for depression alone may not be effective, and an additional step is needed to assess the motivation and health beliefs of patients in order to tailor treatment to the individual. It is unlikely that this latter assessment can be undertaken remotely, and so it may be more prudent to undertake the initial screening in a clinical setting where those who have high depression scores can be seen in a timely manner by the diabetes physician or by the diabetes specialist nurse. Collaboration between physician and nurse in a collaborative systematic care model could be a way to achieve this [57]. Such models have been elaborated in the primary care setting in the Pathways study [58]. In the general hospital setting, a collaborative care model has been developed between diabetes physicians and nurses and the hospital's psychiatric consultation liaison service in the Collaborative Care for Depression Initiative in the Medical setting (CC:DIM) study [59].

7. There should be an agreed policy on the further diagnostic investigation of individuals with a positive test result and on the choices available to those individuals.

Each of the individual screening tools has a threshold above which the risk of depression becomes likely. The diagnosis of depression requires a formal diagnostic interview, and so those who are identified as having a high depression score should be referred promptly to an appropriately trained health care professional who can undertake this interview and offer treatment where the diagnosis of depression is confirmed.

The Treatment

8. There should be an effective treatment or intervention for patients identified through early detection, with evidence of early treatment leading to better outcomes than late treatment.

Until recently, there has been a paucity of evidence about the treatment of depression in people with diabetes, and consequently there has been uncertainty about the most effective and safe way to do so. However, a recent systematic review established that treatment of comorbid major depression and significant depressive symptoms in diabetes is effective, whether psychopharmacological, psychotherapeutical, or collaborative care treatment is provided [6]. Psychological therapies combined with strategies aimed at improving self-management, provided in a specialist setting, showed the largest treatment effects for depression and diabetes [6]. Antidepressant treatment is also effective, but in general antidepressants do not lead to improvements in glycemic control, with the exception of sertraline. The mechanism for the improved glycemic control with sertraline is unknown. Collaborative care provided in the primary care setting showed moderately large effects [6]. As all treatment modalities show considerable effect and patient self-management is of great importance in attaining treatment success, the mode and setting of the treatment should be determined on an individual basis and may involve either psychological therapies or antidepressant medication or a combination of both [6].

Psychological Interventions

The common psychological interventions include cognitive behavioral therapy (CBT), interpersonal therapy (IPT), motivational interviewing, problem solving, counseling, and psychodynamic therapy.

The effectiveness of psychological interventions in people with diabetes has been demonstrated in a systematic review of 25 randomized controlled trials of psychological therapies, mostly CBT. Both psychological distress and glycemic control were improved in people receiving active psychological interventions [60]. A further systemic review of 29 trials and meta-analysis of 21 trials by the same group showed that psychological interventions improved glycated hemoglobin by approximately 0.5% (5 mmol/mol) in children but not in adults [61].

Psychological interventions are most effective when combined with self-management diabetes education, suggesting that it is important to provide the person with diabetes self-management skills as well as the psychological support to use these effectively [6].

Although the psychological benefits of regular exercise have not been studied specifically in people with comorbid diabetes and depression, in the general population, moderate physical activity has been shown to improve mental well-being and is an approved treatment for mild depression [9, 20]. Therefore, it is expected that exercise may also improve depressive symptoms as well as glycemic control in people with diabetes.

Antidepressants

Over the last century, there have been significant developments in the pharmacological treatment of depression. In the last 20 years, the use of tricyclic antidepressants, such as amitriptyline and nortriptyline, has gradually been superseded by the serotonin-specific reuptake inhibitors (SSRIs), such as sertraline, fluoxetine, and citalopram, which are possibly better tolerated and certainly safer in overdose. More recently, serotonin-noradrenaline reuptake inhibitors (SNRIs), such as venlafaxine, and mirtazapine, a tetracyclic antidepressant, have added further therapeutic choices. As long as antidepressants are used in adequate doses, they all have similar efficacy in terms of depression outcomes, and therefore the choice of agent largely reflects the side effect profile, patient preference, and individual response [20].

When a patient does not respond to treatment within 4–6 weeks, an alternative agent, either within class or another class, should be tried instead [20]. Nonresponsive cases and those with marked risk of suicidal behavior will require prompt referral to specialist mental health services. Long-term treatment for 6–24 months is necessary to minimize the risk of relapse.

SSRIs are probably the treatment of choice in people with diabetes because they are less cardiotoxic than tricyclic antidepressants and are safer in overdose. Certain antidepressants, including mirtazapine, paroxetine, and some tricyclic antidepressants may induce significant weight gain and are less suitable as weight gain can worsen insulin resistance and glycemic control [62].

Certain drug interactions should be considered; for example, fluoxetine and sertraline inhibit the enzymes involved in the metabolism of oral diabetes treatment, thereby increasing the risk of hypoglycemia [63].

Although early trials excluded people with diabetes, more recent studies have shown that the response to antidepressants is similar to the general population [6]. Evidence is also emerging that glycemic control may also be improved, although the data are more conflicting. A recent systematic review suggested that sertraline may have specific advantages for glycemic control [6].

There are no long-term studies of the effectiveness of these treatments in terms of the prevention of diabetes complications; however, the benefits in glycemic control, particularly with the psychological interventions, may reasonably be expected to reduce the long-term complication rate.

9. There should be agreed evidence-based policies covering which individuals should be offered treatment and the appropriate treatment to be offered.

There are evidence-based national and international guidelines that give coherent recommendations for the treatment of depression [9, 20].

10. Clinical management of the condition and patient outcomes should be optimized in all health care providers prior to participation in a screening program.

Primary care doctors are routinely involved in the treatment of diabetes and depression and should have the necessary skills to identify and manage these two conditions. However, the number of people with undiagnosed depression would suggest that current health services are not meeting this health demand. In the Netherlands Study of Depression and Anxiety, a cohort study performed in primary care and specialist mental health settings, less than half of participants with depressive or anxiety symptoms who visited their GP and asked for treatment subsequently received adequate guideline-based treatment [64].

The Screening Program

Currently, there are no formalized screening programs for depression in people with diabetes, and therefore most of the remaining criteria are not fulfilled, but nevertheless it is instructive to consider these to gain an understanding of what further research is needed to justify screening. Although some of these criteria are best applied to large national programs, the principles are also important for locally implemented screening.

11. There should be evidence from high quality randomized controlled trials that the screening program is effective in reducing mortality or morbidity.

There have been no randomized controlled trials showing that screening for depression in people with diabetes is effective. The only trial that evaluated a screening program with provision of the results to the individual with diabetes and doctor did not show improvement in health outcomes [55]. Screening will only lead to reduced morbidity or mortality if those identified by screening receive adequate treatment thereafter; however, as people with mental and physical health comorbidity have substantially higher mortality rates, if adequate treatment is provided to those identified by screening and patients are motivated to adhere to treatment, a beneficial effect in terms of mortality may be expected. Further trials are needed to demonstrate this.

12. The complete screening program should be clinically, socially, and ethically acceptable to health professionals and the public.

As formal screening programs are not in place, this has not been assessed. Given the reticence of some patients to embark on intensive treatments, it is possible that a universal screening program would not be acceptable [53]. As such, a screening program may need to be targeted toward high-risk individuals. People with comorbid depression and diabetes are a heterogeneous group, and different people may require different treatment and management.

13. The benefit from the screening program should outweigh the physical and psychological harm.

It is truism that all screening programs cause harm; only some are beneficial and in only a smaller proportion does the benefit outweigh the harm. This is a particular concern if identification of a patient is not followed by proper explanation and provision of effective treatment. The risks and benefits of screening for depression in people with diabetes have not been studied systematically.

14. The screening program should be cost-effective.

The cost-effectiveness of screening for depression has not been formally assessed in research, and indeed these analyses are only possible after the demonstration of clinical effectiveness of a screening procedure followed by treatment. The current challenge is to motivate patients identified by screening for treatment, to provide an effective treatment, and to support the patient in their self-management behaviors.

Most of the currently available questionnaire screening tools are quick and inexpensive, and so if used alone, it is likely that the associated costs will be less than the additional costs of the treatment of depression; however, the increased workload needed to undertake diagnostic interviews in patients identified as case by screening may be considerable, and cost-effectiveness cannot be assumed. If treatment of depression is shown to improve long-term diabetes complications, it is likely that screening and treatment would be cost-effective.

15. There should be a plan for managing and monitoring the screening program and an agreed set of quality assurance standards.

At present, there are no formal screening programs for screening for depression in people with diabetes, and current screening is opportunistic. As such, there is no agreed set of quality assurance standards.

16. Adequate staffing and facilities for testing, diagnosis, treatment, and program management should be available prior to the commencement of the screening program.

Most primary care physicians are responsible for the treatment of diabetes and depression and therefore have the necessary skills to undertake screening for depression in this patient group. Although only 5% of the population has diabetes, the intensive nature of the diagnostic interview may limit the ability to manage people who screen positive, unless a high-risk strategy for screening is adopted.

17. All other options for managing the condition should have been considered (e.g., improving treatment, providing other services) to ensure that no more cost-effective intervention could be introduced or current interventions increased within the resources available.

The evidence would suggest that undiagnosed depression is contributing to significant morbidity in people with diabetes. Although treatment of depression is available for people with diabetes, it can only be offered if the diagnosis is made. As depression to a large extent cannot be prevented, case finding is needed as a prerequisite to treatment. At present, the best model for screening is unknown, but high-risk screening or opportunistic screening is likely to prove more effective than universal screening [57].

18. Evidence-based information, explaining the consequences of testing, investigation, and treatment should be made available to potential participants to assist them in making an informed choice.

National patient and professional groups, such as Diabetes UK and the Dialogue on Diabetes and Depression, have worked to increase awareness about the importance of comorbid depression. Despite this, many patients do not recognize depression as a complication of diabetes and may therefore not avail themselves of self-administered depression screening tools.

19. Public pressure for widening the eligibility criteria for reducing the screening interval and for increasing the sensitivity of the testing process should be anticipated. Decisions about these parameters should be scientifically justifiable to the public.

Most people with diabetes receive an annual assessment of their diabetes management which incorporates a review of diabetes complications. This would provide an opportunity to screen for depression. It seems unlikely that there would be pressure to increase the frequency of this screening, but patients should be encouraged to discuss depressive symptoms if they occur in the interim.

Conclusion

The increased burden of comorbid diabetes and depression provides an imperative to screen for depression in people with diabetes. Most of the criteria relating to the illnesses and their screening tests are fulfilled. Although some of the criteria used to evaluate a screening program are not satisfied, this is largely because formal screening does not take place yet. Although this analysis would suggest that screening for depression in people with diabetes may be worthwhile, further research is needed to determine the optimal way of delivering screening programs and then to demonstrate their clinical and cost-effectiveness.

References

1. Anderson RJ, Freedland KE, Clouse RE, Lustman PJ. The prevalence of comorbid depression in adults with diabetes: a meta-analysis. Diabetes Care. 2001;24(6):1069–78.
2. Hermanns N, Scheff C, Kulzer B, Weyers P, Pauli P, Kubiak T, et al. Association of glucose levels and glucose variability with mood in type 1 diabetic patients. Diabetologia. 2007;50(5):930–3.
3. Jacobson AM, Samson JA, Weinger K, Ryan CM. Diabetes, the brain, and behavior: is there a biological mechanism underlying the association between diabetes and depression? Int Rev Neurobiol. 2002;51:455–79.
4. de Groot M, Anderson R, Freedland KE, Clouse RE, Lustman PJ. Association of depression and diabetes complications: a meta-analysis. Psychosom Med. 2001;63(4):619–30.
5. Goldney RD, Phillips PJ, Fisher LJ, Wilson DH. Diabetes, depression, and quality of life: a population study. Diabetes Care. 2004;27(5):1066–70.
6. van der Feltz-Cornelis CM, Nuyen J, Stoop C, Chan J, Jacobson AM, Katon W, et al. Effect of interventions for major depressive disorder and significant depressive symptoms in patients with diabetes mellitus: a systematic review and meta-analysis. Gen Hosp Psychiatry. 2010;32(4):380–95.
7. Egede LE, Ellis C. Diabetes and depression: global perspectives. In: IDF diabetes atlas. Brussels: International Diabetes Federation; 2009. p. 1–21.
8. American Diabetes Association. Executive summary: standards of medical care in diabetes – 2011. Diabetes Care. 2011;34 Suppl 1:S4–10.
9. National Collaborating Centre for Mental Health. Depression in adults with a chronic physical health problem. London: The British Psychological Society and The Royal College of Psychiatrists; 2010.
10. UK National Screening Committee. Criteria for appraising the viability, effectiveness and appropriateness of a screening programme. 2011. http://www.screening.nhs.uk/criteria. Accessed 15 Nov 2011.
11. Whiting DR, Guariguata L, Weil C, Shaw J. IDF diabetes atlas: global estimates of the prevalence of diabetes for 2011 and 2030. Diabetes Res Clin Pract. 2011;94(3):311–21.
12. Sicree R, Shaw J, Zimmett P. The global burden: diabetes and impaired glucose tolerance. In: IDF diabetes atlas. Brussels: International Diabetes Federation; 2009. p. 1–105.
13. Roglic G, Unwin N. Mortality attributable to diabetes: estimates for the year 2010. Diabetes Res Clin Pract. 2010;87(1):15–9.
14. Intensive blood-glucose control with sulphonylureas or insulin compared with conventional treatment and risk of complications in patients with type 2 diabetes (UKPDS 33). UK Prospective Diabetes Study (UKPDS) Group. Lancet. 1998;352(9131):837–53.
15. Murray CJ, Lopez AD. Alternative projections of mortality and disability by cause 1990–2020: global burden of disease study. Lancet. 1997;349(9064):1498–504.
16. American Psychiatric Association. Diagnostic and statistical manual of mental disorders. 4th ed. Washington: American Psychiatric Association; 1994.
17. Rugulies R. Depression as a predictor for coronary heart disease. A review and meta-analysis. Am J Prev Med. 2002;23(1):51–61.
18. Meijer A, Conradi HJ, Bos EH, Thombs BD, van Melle JP, de Jonge JP. Prognostic association of depression following myocardial infarction with mortality and cardiovascular events: a meta-analysis of 25 years of research. Gen Hosp Psychiatry. 2011;33(3):203–16.
19. Berto P, D'Ilario D, Ruffo P, Di VR, Rizzo F. Depression: cost-of-illness studies in the international literature, a review. J Ment Health Policy Econ. 2000;3(1):3–10.
20. National Collaborating Centre for Mental Health. Common mental health disorders: identification and pathways to care CG123. London: National Institute of Health and Clinical Excellence; 2011.
21. van der Feltz-Cornelis CM, Ten Have M. Penninx BW, Beekman AT, Smit JH, de Graaf R. Presence of comorbid somatic disorders among patients referred to mental health care in the Netherlands. Psychiatr Serv. 2010;61(11):1119–25.

22. Colton CW, Manderscheid RW. Congruencies in increased mortality rates, years of potential life lost, and causes of death among public mental health clients in eight states. Prev Chronic Dis. 2006;3(2):A42.
23. Hermanns N, Kulzer B, Krichbaum M, Kubiak T, Haak T. Affective and anxiety disorders in a German sample of diabetic patients: prevalence, comorbidity and risk factors. Diabet Med. 2005;22(3):293–300.
24. Nouwen A, Winkley K, Twisk J, Lloyd CE, Peyrot M, Ismail K, et al. Type 2 diabetes mellitus as a risk factor for the onset of depression: a systematic review and meta-analysis. Diabetologia. 2010;53(12):2480–6.
25. Ludman EJ, Katon W, Russo J, Von KM, Simon G, Ciechanowski P, et al. Depression and diabetes symptom burden. Gen Hosp Psychiatry. 2004;26(6):430–6.
26. Ciechanowski PS, Katon WJ, Russo JE. Depression and diabetes: impact of depressive symptoms on adherence, function, and costs. Arch Intern Med. 2000;160(21):3278–85.
27. Hislop AL, Fegan PG, Schlaeppi MJ, Duck M, Yeap BB. Prevalence and associations of psychological distress in young adults with type 1 diabetes. Diabet Med. 2008;25(1):91–6.
28. Aikens JE, Perkins DW, Piette JD, Lipton B. Association between depression and concurrent type 2 diabetes outcomes varies by diabetes regimen. Diabet Med. 2008;25(11):1324–9.
29. Lin EH, Rutter CM, Katon W, Heckbert SR, Ciechanowski P, Oliver MM, et al. Depression and advanced complications of diabetes: a prospective cohort study. Diabetes Care. 2010;33(2):264–9.
30. Lin EH, Heckbert SR, Rutter CM, Katon WJ, Ciechanowski P, Ludman EJ, et al. Depression and increased mortality in diabetes: unexpected causes of death. Ann Fam Med. 2009;7(5):414–21.
31. Egede LE, Zheng D, Simpson K. Comorbid depression is associated with increased health care use and expenditures in individuals with diabetes. Diabetes Care. 2002;25(3):464–70.
32. Stratton IM, Adler AI, Neil HA, Matthews DR, Manley SE, Cull CA, et al. Association of glycaemia with macrovascular and microvascular complications of type 2 diabetes (UKPDS 35): prospective observational study. BMJ. 2000;321(7258):405–12.
33. Currie CJ, Peters JR, Tynan A, Evans M, Heine RJ, Bracco OL, et al. Survival as a function of HbA(1c) in people with type 2 diabetes: a retrospective cohort study. Lancet. 2010;375(9713): 481–9.
34. The effect of intensive treatment of diabetes on the development and progression of long-term complications in insulin-dependent diabetes mellitus. The Diabetes Control and Complications Trial Research Group. N Engl J Med. 1993;329(14):977–86.
35. Holman RR, Paul SK, Bethel MA, Matthews DR, Neil HA. 10-year follow-up of intensive glucose control in type 2 diabetes. N Engl J Med. 2008;359(15):1577–89.
36. Nathan DM, Cleary PA, Backlund JY, Genuth SM, Lachin JM, Orchard TJ, et al. Intensive diabetes treatment and cardiovascular disease in patients with type 1 diabetes. N Engl J Med. 2005;353(25):2643–53.
37. Gerstein HC, Miller ME, Genuth S, Ismail-Beigi F, Buse JB, Goff Jr DC, et al. Long-term effects of intensive glucose lowering on cardiovascular outcomes. N Engl J Med. 2011;364(9):818–28.
38. Gerstein HC, Miller ME, Byington RP, Goff Jr DC, Bigger JT, Buse JB, et al. Effects of intensive glucose lowering in type 2 diabetes. N Engl J Med. 2008;358(24):2545–59.
39. Patel A, Macmahon S, Chalmers J, Neal B, Billot L, Woodward M, et al. Intensive blood glucose control and vascular outcomes in patients with type 2 diabetes. N Engl J Med. 2008;358(24):2560–72.
40. Duckworth W, Abraira C, Moritz T, Reda D, Emanuele N, Reaven PD, et al. Glucose control and vascular complications in veterans with type 2 diabetes. N Engl J Med. 2009;360(2): 129–39.
41. Kovacs M, Mukerji P, Drash A, Iyengar S. Biomedical and psychiatric risk factors for retinopathy among children with IDDM. Diabetes Care. 1995;18(12):1592–9.
42. Cohen ST, Welch G, Jacobson AM, de Groot M, Samson J. The association of lifetime psychiatric illness and increased retinopathy in patients with type I diabetes mellitus. Psychosomatics. 1997;38(2):98–108.

43. Polonsky WH, Anderson BJ, Lohrer PA, Welch G, Jacobson AM, Aponte JE, et al. Assessment of diabetes-related distress. Diabetes Care. 1995;18(6):754–60.
44. Meeuwissen JA, van der Feltz-Cornelis CM, van Marwijk HW, Rijnders PB, Donker MC. A stepped care programme for depression management: an uncontrolled pre-post study in primary and secondary care in the Netherlands. Int J Integr Care. 2008;8:e05.
45. Robins LN, Wing J, Wittchen HU, Helzer JE, Babor TF, Burke J, et al. The composite international diagnostic interview. An epidemiologic Instrument suitable for use in conjunction with different diagnostic systems and in different cultures. Arch Gen Psychiatry. 1988;45(12):1069–77.
46. Amorim P, Lecrubier Y, Weiller E, Hergueta T, Sheehan D. DSM-IH-R psychotic disorders: procedural validity of the mini international neuropsychiatric interview (MINI). Concordance and causes for discordance with the CIDI. Eur Psychiatry. 1998;13(1):26–34.
47. Beck AT, Ward CH, Mendelson M, Mock J, Erbaugh J. An inventory for measuring depression. Arch Gen Psychiatry. 1961;4:561–71.
48. Radloff LS. The CES-D scale: a self report depression scale for research in the general population. Appl Psychol Meas. 1977;1:385–401.
49. Spitzer RL, Kroenke K, Williams JB. Validation and utility of a self-report version of PRIME-MD: the PHQ primary care study. Primary Care Evaluation of Mental Disorders. Patient Health Questionnaire. JAMA. 1999;282(18):1737–44.
50. Roy T, Lloyd CE, Pouwer F, Holt RI, Sartorius N. Screening tools used for measuring depression among people with type 1 and type 2 diabetes: a systematic review. Diabet Med. 2012; 29(2):164–75.
51. Zigmond AS, Snaith RP. The hospital anxiety and depression scale. Acta Psychiatr Scand. 1983;67(6):361–70.
52. Kroenke K, Spitzer RL, Williams JB, Lowe B. The patient health questionnaire somatic, anxiety, and depressive symptom scales: a systematic review. Gen Hosp Psychiatry. 2010;32(4):345–59.
53. van Steenbergen-Weijenburg KM, de Vroege L, Ploeger RR, Brals JW, Vloedbeld MG, Veneman TF, et al. Validation of the PHQ-9 as a screening instrument for depression in diabetes patients in specialized outpatient clinics. BMC Health Serv Res. 2010;10:235.
54. Whooley MA, Avins AL, Miranda J, Browner WS. Case-finding instruments for depression. Two questions are as good as many. J Gen Intern Med. 1997;12(7):439–45.
55. Pouwer F, Tack CJ, Geelhoed-Duijvestijn PH, Bazelmans E, Beekman AT, Heine RJ, et al. Limited effect of screening for depression with written feedback in outpatients with diabetes mellitus: a randomised controlled trial. Diabetologia. 2011;54(4):741–8.
56. Gilbody S, Sheldon T, House A. Screening and case-finding instruments for depression: a meta-analysis. CMAJ. 2008;178(8):997–1003.
57. van der Feltz-Cornelis CM. Depression in diabetes mellitus: to screen or not to screen? A patient-centred approach. Br J Diab Vasc Dis. 2011;11(6):276–81.
58. Katon WJ, Von Korff M, Lin EH, Simon G, Ludman E, Russo J, et al. The pathways study: a randomized trial of collaborative care in patients with diabetes and depression. Arch Gen Psychiatry. 2004;61(10):1042–9.
59. Horn EK, van Benthem TB, Hakkaart-van RL, van Marwijk HW, Beekman AT, Rutten FF, et al. Cost-effectiveness of collaborative care for chronically ill patients with comorbid depressive disorder in the general hospital setting, a randomised controlled trial. BMC Health Serv Res. 2007;7:28.
60. Ismail K, Winkley K, Rabe-Hesketh S. Systematic review and meta-analysis of randomised controlled trials of psychological interventions to improve glycaemic control in patients with type 2 diabetes. Lancet. 2004;363(9421):1589–97.
61. Winkley K, Ismail K, Landau S, Eisler I. Psychological interventions to improve glycaemic control in patients with type 1 diabetes: systematic review and meta-analysis of randomised controlled trials. BMJ. 2006;333(7558):65.
62. Serretti A, Mandelli L. Antidepressants and body weight: a comprehensive review and meta-analysis. J Clin Psychiatry. 2010;71(10):1259–72.

63. Pollak PT, Mukherjee SD, Fraser AD. Sertraline-induced hypoglycemia. Ann Pharmacother. 2001;35(11):1371–4.
64. Smolders M, Laurant M, Verhaak P, Prins M, van Marwijk H, Penninx B, et al. Adherence to evidence-based guidelines for depression and anxiety disorders is associated with recording of the diagnosis. Gen Hosp Psychiatry. 2009;31(5):460–9.

Chapter 4
Cultural Applicability of Screening Tools for Measuring Symptoms of Depression

Tapash Roy and Cathy E. Lloyd

Abstract Both the type as well as the severity of depressive symptoms requires assessment through culturally sensitive screening tools, if appropriate psychological services are to be provided. Awareness of culturally appropriate terminology for depression is a useful way of bridging the gap between lay and biomedical models of illness and may help improve levels of recognition, measurement, and treatment. In this chapter, the cultural meaning of depression, issues concerning culturally appropriate translations, and the cultural applicability of depression screening tools, in those whose main language is not English, will be discussed and reflected upon. This chapter will also illustrate the relevance of a culture-centered approach to our understanding of mental health illness and will outline some of the key issues related to the development of culturally sensitive depression screening tools to be used in South Asians.

Keywords Depression • Measurement • Screening tools • Cultural applicability Minority ethnic groups • South Asians

T. Roy, MBBS, M.Sc., Ph.D. (✉)
Division of Social Research in Medicines and Health,
The University of Nottingham, Nottingham, UK
e-mail: tapash_68@hotmail.com

C.E. Lloyd, Ph.D.
Faculty of Health and Social Care, The Open University,
Buckinghamshire, UK
e-mail: cathy.lloyd@open.ac.uk

C.E. Lloyd et al. (eds.), *Screening for Depression and Other Psychological Problems in Diabetes*,
DOI 10.1007/978-0-85729-751-8_4, © Springer-Verlag London 2013

Introduction

People with type 2 diabetes are known to have an increased risk of developing mental health problems, including depression, anxiety, and other forms of emotional and psychological distress [1]. Further to its implications for physical, mental, and social well-being, depression contributes to poor diabetes self-care, diminished quality of life, and higher rates of medical morbidity and mortality, as well as increased healthcare costs [2–5]. However, in spite of the huge impact of comorbid depression and diabetes on the individual and its importance as a public health problem, little is known about the existence of psychological problems in South Asians living with diabetes [6]. There is increasing recognition that culture plays a significant role in shaping depressive symptoms, its awareness and interpretation, and care-seeking. But little is written about screening for these conditions within a cultural perspective. It appears that the incidence and prevalence of health problems vary among people of different cultural backgrounds due to the interplay of biological, psychological, and social factors [7]. In groups whose main language is not English, including migrants such as those from South Asian communities living in the UK, or those from non-Western societies, there are serious limitations to the research that has been carried out to date in depression and diabetes [8–10]. In order to build upon and improve research, it helps to learn lessons from past experiences in this field. In this regard, both the type as well as the severity of depressive symptoms requires assessment through culturally appropriate screening tools, if appropriate psychological services are to be provided. In this chapter, the cultural meaning of depression, issues concerning culturally appropriate translations, and the applicability of two depression screening tools (the Patient Health Questionnaire and World Health Organization Well-Being Questionnaire), in those whose main language is not English, will be discussed and reflected upon. More specifically, we will consider two pieces of our recent research with Bangladeshis, and our experiences in carrying out these studies will be used to inform the debate around how we can develop valid and culturally tailored depression screening tools for populations with high illiteracy rates.

Cultural Sensitivity: Theoretical Perspectives

The term "culture" is often misused or overused. In its early anthropologic era, culture referred to the set of shared attitudes, values, and practices that characterize social groups. It therefore emerged as a concept encompassing all human phenomena that are not purely the result of human genetics. This usage tended to represent cultures as bounded, fixed entities, neglecting crucial differences among and within groups, and it risked reducing culture to an autonomous variable among others [11]. But in fact, culture is not a thing which can be calculated as a statistical variable; it is a process by which day-to-day activities acquire emotional and moral meaning for people. As Kleinman ([11]: pp. 952) highlighted, "cultural processes include the embodiment of meaning in habitual and physiological reactions, the understanding of what are at stake in particular situations, the development of interpersonal relationships, religious practices, and the cultivation of collective and individual identity. Treating culture as a fixed variable rather than as a concept seriously impedes our ability to understand and respond to disease states such as depression."

The debate on the complex links between culture, health, and social and psychological well-being is only now beginning to be explored globally [12–16]. The recent focus of interest in culture as an important determinant in psychiatric research emerges with huge demographic change in the ethnic composition of many Western countries. A culturally sensitive approach to health care has therefore emerged that considers ethnic minorities' particular requirements within a health system. This approach emphasizes providing minorities with the same sort of health service as mainstream society but at the same time takes into account the cultural "diversities" of the minority groups. Furthermore, "etic" and "emic" views are captured by the researchers to explain differences in mental health [17]. In particular, this debate has focused on the theoretical basis of the "etic" and "emic" approaches which emphasize either biological universality or cultural diversity, respectively, as discussed below.

An "etic" approach focuses on the perceptions of professionals and assumes that mental health problems as conceptualized by a biomedically driven psychiatry hence are automatically valid in any settings. This approach underpins the bulk of epidemiological research worldwide, particularly in Western industrialized countries. In contrast, an "emic" approach is based on acknowledging the perceptions of the local community. Each of these perspectives is quite distinctive, but in reality they also overlap. This effort of acknowledging and incorporating the profound role played by culture in the experience, expression, diagnosis, and management of mental illness had a significant role in the development of medical anthropology in health care, particularly in developing countries [14]. Anthropologists have extensively discussed a major difference among illness explanatory models, i.e., the physical framework that attributes illness to physical causes and the psychosocial framework that attributes illness to thoughts and emotions, usually resulting from social factors [18].

Measuring depression across cultures has always been a source of controversy. Studies in the UK report ethnic and cultural variations in the presentation, general practitioners' assessment, and management of common mental health problems [15, 19–21]. When it comes to the question of using depression screening instruments, "emic" instruments are those developed in the culture in which they are to be used, and "etic" ones are developed in one culture but used without reservation in other cultures [22]. Most research still use "etic" instruments, despite the criticism that one cannot apply diagnostic or other research instruments developed in one culture to subjects who live in another culture [23].

Kleinman [23] called for a new "cross-cultural" psychiatry that accounts for local meanings and related behaviors in order to improve the assessment of psychological morbidity and its treatment. He argued that the application of instruments developed in one culture to measure psychological distress in another possibly will generate misleading information [23]. Patel [14] explained that an important drawback in cross-cultural psychiatry is that it is a highly specialized area of interest to researchers and academics, particularly in industrialized countries, and that the majority of the research in nonindustrialized countries often follows the "etic" approach where "culture" is rarely considered as a determinant. He further highlighted that whereas Western societies are considered "multicultural" so that studies need to be conducted for different ethnic groups to ensure the findings are "culturally sensitive and correct," nonindustrialized societies are not offered the same privilege ([14]: pp. 34). As suggested by Bhui and Bhugra [15], a popular approach to address these concerns is to use an existing instrument and modify it in the light of ethnographic work looking at local cultural perspectives of illness under study.

This debate around two epistemological approaches within cross-cultural psychiatry has prompted researchers to adapt a more flexible approach in considering local realities. In order to overcome the limitations of both these approaches, researchers have recently attempted to combine quantitative research with an approach which uses local narratives and explanatory models of mental health problems [17, 24, 25]. Bhui [26] suggested that epidemiologists need to learn more about qualitative data analysis, its use with quantitative data, and the limitations of each approach [15, 26]. At this point, one might wonder what should be the validity criteria for a study that combines both types of methods. Im et al. [27] argued that there are criteria that can be applied to both quantitative and qualitative cross-cultural research. These include not only cultural relevance, contextuality, and appropriateness but also mutual respect and flexibility in approach. The use of two or more different data collection methods (often termed "triangulation"), where the findings are compared and integrated, has indeed proved useful in gaining insights into the research question from different perspectives.

Cultural Meanings of Depression

Evidence suggests that the prevalence of depressive disorders may differ between countries and within countries and across various ethnicities [28]. Moreover, depression in individuals is known to be influenced by social and cultural factors; hence, it is likely that the occurrence of depression will vary among and within societies [29]. In a recent empirical research study examining ethnic differences in depression in people with diabetes in the UK, South Asians reported lower levels of diagnosed depressive disorder compared with their Caucasian counterparts [30]. However, the authors noted that this may have been due to differences in either the presentation of symptoms or a lack of cultural appropriateness of Western methods of identifying depression. Similarly, Bhui et al. [31], in a survey in London with Punjabi and English general practice attendees, reported that the Punjabis were not rated as having more depression than the English participants, but they did have more depressive ideas. Therefore, the measurement of depression and its association with diabetes must also be assessed within different cultural settings. Although the association between depression and diabetes has been found consistently, the transcultural validity of these findings remains to be shown.

Table 4.1 Summary: the ADCAD-DS in the UK

This study aimed to develop culturally competent translations (in both written and audio formats) of two screening tools used to measure symptoms of depression in languages with no written form and attempted to establish their face validity
Adults with type 2 diabetes from two South Asian minority ethnic groups (from Bangladesh and Pakistan) whose main language is only spoken (Sylheti and Mirpuri) were recruited via the Birmingham Heartlands Hospital Diabetes Centre. Participants attended two focus group meetings to consider the content and method of delivery of two questionnaires measuring symptoms of depression, the Patient Health Questionnaire (PHQ-9) and the World Health Organization Well-Being Index (WHO-5)
Culturally equivalent content was achieved for both questionnaires in both languages. The Mirpuri men and women groups did not indicate a clear preference for either mode of questionnaire delivery; however the Sylheti groups' preference was for independent audio delivery in their spoken language
This study established the face validity of the PHQ-9 and the WHO-5 for Sylheti and Mirpuri speakers in an audio delivery format and called for further validation and psychometric testing in order to determine the feasibility of wider use among minority ethnic populations

The Alternative Data Collection in Asians with Diabetes – Depression Study (ADCAD-DS) was designed to develop culturally appropriate methods for administering and collecting reliable and valid data on psychological morbidity in South Asian people with type 2 diabetes (specifically Mirpuri and Sylheti speakers). The key findings from this study are illustrated in Table 4.1. Two questionnaires were considered, the Patient Health Questionnaire (PHQ-9) and the World Health Organization Well-Being Questionnaire (WHO-5), by individuals with type 2 diabetes from two minority ethnic populations living in Birmingham, so that accurate and culturally sensitive written and spoken translations could be developed.

During the course of this study, participants attended a series of focus group sessions and discussed the concept of depression and the use and cultural equivalency of the terms used in these two questionnaires, as well as the two standard questions currently used in general practice in the UK for depression screening [10]. A further study was carried out in Bangladesh with a bigger sample of Bengali and Sylheti speakers to validate the cultural applicability of these newly developed tools. The Bangladesh study used a one-to-one data collection technique. This discussion specifically focuses on our experience with Bangladeshis (both in the UK and at their origin in Bangladesh).

During the focus group sessions with Sylheti speakers in the UK and in the one-to-one interviews with Bengali and Sylheti speakers in Bangladesh, participants were asked whether they recognized terms such as "depressed," "cheerful," and "feeling down" and were asked to consider the meaning these terms had in their culture. The Bengali and Sylheti alternatives for the actual content of the two standard questions and the PHQ-9 and WHO-5 questionnaires were discussed and recommendations for any suggested changes made. This participatory discussion helped the development process of culturally equivalent translated written and audio versions of the questionnaires [10].

Participants from both study sites were clear that they understood what feeling depressed or feeling low meant to them. However, a range of local terms and descriptions were used to express their understanding of the concept of depression, which

Table 4.2 Local terms for depression

UK study: Sylheti speakers	Bangladesh study: Sylheti speakers	Bangladesh study: Bengali speakers
Duschinta (worry)	*Duschinta* (worry)	*Duschinta* (worry)
Mon bejar (bad mood)	*Chinta rog* (worry illness)	*Chinta rog* (worry illness)
Mon mora (sadness)	*Mon bejar* (bad mood)	*Mon kharap* (bad mood)
Mon bala nay (not in good mood)	*Mon mora* (sadness)	*Mon var* (pressure on the mind)
Tension (anxiety)	*Mathaye tension* (tension on my head)	*Tension* (anxiety)
Dorod (paid)	*Dorod* (pain)	*Tension rog* (anxiety illness)
Shorir durbol (tiredness)	*Matha var* (weight on my head)	*Durbolota* (weakness/tiredness)
Matha var (weight on my head)	*Buk var* (weight on my heart)	*Beytha* (pain)
Buk var (weight on the heart)	*Shanti nai* (joylessness)	*Matha var* (weight on the head)
Shanti nai (joylessness)	Mental	*Matha nosto* (going mad)
Mental case	*Manoshik rog* (mental disorder)	*Orthonoitik chap* (financial tension)
Off mood		*Mathaye tension* (tension on the head)
		Buk dhorfor (palpitation)
		Buk var (weight on the chest)
		Hai hutash (grievances)
		Manoshik chap (mental pressure)

are summarized in an ascending order in Table 4.2. The participants also described a wide range of physical, emotional, and social problems as manifestations of depression. In the Sylheti groups, the terms used for the symptoms of depression translated into English as "worry" or "bad mood" or "off mood" or "pain/sadness" or "weight on my heart/mind" or "joylessness" and even tiredness. In addition to these, the Bengali speakers further mentioned "weight on the head" or "tension on the head" or "palpitation" or "weight on the chest" and "grievances" as manifestations of depression. In both groups, somatization was fairly common, and depression was often described in terms of somatic symptoms or physical pain.

We have considered these findings according to the Herdman et al. [32] criteria for achieving conceptual and item equivalence. Firstly, in terms of conceptual equivalence, our findings suggest that the concept of depression may not have universal meaning and that there are alternative ways to describe depressive symptomatology. Even within Bangladesh, meanings and expression of depression differed significantly between Bengali and Sylheti speakers. In those individuals who took part in our research, depression was frequently described in terms of somatic symptoms, some of which may also overlap with the symptoms of diabetes. Some research has suggested that there may be a particular "language of emotions" in certain ethnic groups, which might be more related to the somatic symptoms of depression or psychological distress, and these have often been ignored in attempts to measure depressive symptomatology [33, 34].

These variations in symptoms and ways to describe depressive symptomatology can be seen as culturally influenced [10]. Earlier studies suggested that somatization (the process by which psychological distress is "converted" to somatic symptoms) was the cultural equivalent of depression, typically occurring in non-Western cultures [14]. There is from now growing evidence studies in primary and general health-care settings that somatic symptoms are common presenting features of depression throughout the world regardless of cultural background [10, 35–39]. The terms "anxiety" and "depression" as used in English both have basically somatic roots [16]. However, reporting somatic symptoms depends on how somatization is defined cross-culturally [38].

It is now well recognized that the cultural background of a person is likely to determine whether depression will be experienced and expressed in psychological and emotional terms, or in physical terms [40]. In many cultures, depressed patients, especially in the initial phase, will not complain about a disposition to depression. There is an assumption that people from traditional cultures may not distinguish between the emotions of anxiety, irritability, and depression because they tend to express distress in somatic terms [41] or they may organize their concepts of emotional well-being in ways different from Western ones [10, 16, 39]. Some of these conditions may be universal and some are culturally distinct, but all are meaningful within particular cultural contexts. Therefore, it is important to understand the local term(s) and the popular concepts of the causes, effects of particular health problems, and help seeking in the community if communication is to be improved between patients and health-care providers [42, 43].

Indeed, patients and their families may have their own ideas about the illness as opposed to clinicians' views. Research among South Asian populations has shown that patients with depression usually link their depressive symptoms to different causes, for example, any upsetting conditions, accidents or daily occurrence of events, unfavorable living conditions, financial problems, or physical illness, and therefore consider it as a natural occurrence [31, 35, 36, 39]. Bhugra and Mastrogianni ([16]: pp.16) termed this somatization, in a South Asian culture, could reflect "suffering and dependency needs, while disguising the affective aspects of common mental disorder." However, in other cultures too, for example, in Arabic populations, patients use a variety of somatic descriptions to express the meanings of depression [44] and often associate depression with aches, pains, and weakness [45]. The term "depression" itself is often absent from the languages of many cultures or rarely used [39, 44, 46], or it is construed differently [10, 16, 47]. As the meaning of depression changes as a result of cultural and geographical influence and somatization of symptoms is very common, it is crucial to consider these issues while developing culturally sensitive depression measurement instruments.

Translation Dilemmas in Cross-Cultural Research

Translating concepts across culture is crucial in order to develop culturally appropriate measurement tools, diagnosis, and services for depression. During the questionnaire development process of our research in the UK, we used forward and backward translation techniques. Any discrepancies in the back translation were discussed and a final version agreed by the two translators and the researchers, which we consider as an essential step to achieve cultural accuracy and/or equivalency. In this section, we will reflect upon our experiences with translation issues during the process of instrument development for our studies in South Asian people living in Birmingham, UK.

It is fundamental that the act of translation/interpretation is explored and that the epistemological implications of being the researcher and/or translator/interpreter at the same time are examined. The debate on translation and interpretation in research should involve the hierarchies of language, power, and the situated epistemologies of the researcher and issues around naming and speaking for people who may be seen as "other." In any setting, individuals who do not speak the dominant language of the international research arena need to depend on others to speak for them; "speaking for others, in any language is a critical issue, which involves the use of language to construct self and other" ([48]: pp. 167). During our focus group sessions with Sylheti individuals in Birmingham, it was noted that participants raised their concern about the utility of interpreters used in doctors' consultations:

> Sometimes I have to use interpreters during consultations. I did not find even interpreters explaining things to me properly. They just translate things, I believe – they will ask me something in Sylheti that the GP wants to know and then will translate that back to the GP in a language that I don't understand at all. I actually don't know what is going on in between… or even if they are translating my right feelings to the GP (Sylheti woman).

This concern has important implications for any research that uses interpreters or translators. Vyas et al. [49] suggested that, even when interpreters are used to collect data for research studies, the way the information is collected is still a crucial issue. While the translations were seen to have been technically accurate, and also culturally sensitive, the content of the questionnaires and the actual mode of data collection were often seen as inappropriate by both those collecting the data as well as those providing the data (i.e., the study participants).

Such concern indicates a need for participatory research through ensuring participants' involvement with the research process. Participatory research is not without its difficulties however, and its use in studies of community participation in health has sometimes been problematic. Although the principles of community participation have long been operationalized in the developing world as part of the movement for social justice [50], in the UK, the discrepancies between perceived levels of skill, knowledge, or expertise between professional groups and lay members of the community can lead to difficulties in research [51]. Johnson [52] is clear when he describes the only real involvement of lay members of (ethnic minority) user groups is often as being in the role of fieldworkers or research staff, employed because of their ability to speak a particular language or to gain access to certain groups. Real partnerships between health researchers and members of minority ethnic groups in research are rarely cited and seem to be few.

Whether we are the researcher, the translator, or the interpreter, it is important that we situate and engage with these issues because they relate to our own epistemological positions and how we translate cultural concepts and differences across languages and how accurately we represent others. The importance of identifying the act of translation and interpretation is particularly important in terms of exploring our epistemological position as the researchers. While reading through various cross-cultural research studies, it seems that a discussion of the epistemological and methodological issues around translation and interpretation across languages has been neglected in this research field. An explanation for this neglect could be because of the status of the languages involved in the research, the status of the speakers of such languages, and the hierarchy of the languages. As Temple and Young ([48]: pp. 167) explain, "translation itself has power to reinforce or to subvert longstanding cross-cultural relationships but that power tends to rest in how translation is executed and integrated into research design and not just in the act of translation per se."

A recent systematic review of the process of translation and adaptation of health-related quality of life measures suggested that there is currently a misguided preoccupation with the scales being used rather than a focus on the actual concepts being scaled, with too much reliance on unsubstantiated claims of conceptual equivalence [53]. When questionnaires are translated, it is frequently the case that any cultural differences are not accounted for [54–56]. One might argue that both the content and the design of the instrument are equally important, although success in either aspect cannot be fully achieved if the specific needs of the target population are not addressed. In this case, the need for assisted completion or finding other ways of collecting data which does not involve having to complete questionnaires in a written form appears to be crucial. A further consideration must surely be who should be involved in research and how members of minority ethnic communities can participate more fully in research in order to prevent excluding certain sections of the population.

It has become a common trend that when reading through literature on depression screening, little reference is made to language issues, translation, and interpretation or even identification of the process of translation and interpretation, and when reading interview data, the informants all seem fluent English speakers. In this sort of research, the reader might find themselves entirely lost in terms of understanding the research process, the language used to collect, and later interpret the data. As readers, we might find it very difficult to engage with such texts, particularly when there is no available information on the research process and the source language or where the languages of the research are seen as being obstacles that have been overcome and controlled. This is a type of research where the researcher collects data and presents it as a collection of facts from the informants and where the translator and interpreter, the act of translation and interpretation, and the identity of the researcher are seen to be irrelevant to the representation of the informants and to the informants' engagements with that representation [48].

It is important that as researchers we acknowledge our locations within the social world and explore how our locations influence the way we see things. Temple and Young suggest that "there is no neutral position from which to translate" ([48]: pp. 164); therefore the power relationships within research need to be acknowledged, whether it is the relationship between the researcher and informants or between researcher and translator/interpreter. Researchers and academics with an interest in the power of the written word and the process by which it is produced have argued that there is no single correct translation/interpretation of a text, acknowledging the fact that translation is not about synonym, syntax, and definitely not a matter of finding the meaning of a text in a culture by using a dictionary, but in understanding that the language is "tied to local realities, to literacy forms and to changing identities" ([57]: pp. 137).

Through our own experiences in translation and interpretation of data, we have come to learn that communication across languages involves more than a literal transfer of information because the participants, translator, and interpreter are all involved in discussing concepts, ideas, and positions which are all important parts of the negotiation process of getting to grips with "cultural meaning" and "cultural differences." Dictionaries are not sufficient in trying to establish an understanding across languages. Language involves values, beliefs, concepts, and thoughts, which may not have the same conceptual equivalence in the language into which it is to be translated. During translation and interpretation, researchers have to make decisions about the cultural meanings which language carries and spend a lot of time trying to evaluate the degree to which different worlds inhabit the same meaning. In a similar way to a researcher, a translator and interpreter has to position himself/herself actively in the process and is accountable to the way he/she represents the informants and their culture and languages. In our current studies, we have worked with multilingual researchers fluent in the languages of our informants; the researchers have opportunities in terms of research methods that may not necessarily be open to other researchers in cross-cultural research. The researchers are able to discuss points in texts where they had to stop and think about the meaning, and a discussion of the translation/interpretation process became a kind of check on the validity of interpretation [58]. This by no means produces texts that are "absolute truths" because as researchers we are always situated in complex social locations.

Through a dual role as researcher and translator/interpreter, the role seemed to be shifting, and this was linked to how we are positioned. Researching from inside the language of the informants is an emancipatory and epistemological position that Ladd ([59]: pp. 186) suggests "can only be fulfilled by the researcher-translator/interpreter who shares the common culture of those researched." This however does not necessarily mean that the multilingual researcher produces better research than the monolingual researcher, but rather is as an added advantage of our studies. There is an argument that being multilingual is not enough to enable the researchers to "represent others" because translation and interpretation is not just about "racial matching" of researcher with informants; as Twine [60] points out, race and ethnicity are not the only, or always the, overriding factors in translation/interpretation work. In addition to being multilingual and having a certain degree of insiderness, the researcher's position may not be as unproblematic as expected, and as Twine ([60]: pp. 16) further argues, "difference may be a stimulator as well as a block to communication." However, in our case, it worked as a stimulator to fully engage with the informants.

In research where translators and interpreters are employed, it is important to consider whether the translator or interpreter is playing the role of an informant or a "neutral and objective transmitter of messages" ([48]: pp. 167). Without an open dialogue with the translator and interpreter about their views and perceptions of the issues being discussed, it becomes difficult to allow for differences in understanding of words, concepts, and worldviews across languages. Hence, it is important that we report the translator and interpreter's involvement in the research process, since they have also contributed to the knowledge being produced and they are also socially positioned; this would also mean extending calls for reflexivity in cross-cultural research with translators and interpreters.

As individuals, we are all positioned differently in the social world, and so we begin to understand people as social actors. Because we are positioned differently, there is not one way in which to describe our social worlds, but many different ways. Our social locations influence our experiences and the way we describe these experiences. Young [61] argues that as researchers, informants, and translators and interpreters, we are all products of dispositioned accounts. We all have different stories to tell and different histories, and we occupy different social and cultural positions, but we understand each other across difference through dialogue [61].

As researchers, we need to place such perspectives into wider contexts and consider the consequences for the production of research accounts. This means being explicit about our own social, cultural, and political positions, making visible the translation and interpretation process and being "accountable," in addition to including translators and interpreter in debates on reflexivity. Through our research, we have come to learn that one cannot assume that there are no problems in translating cultural concepts across languages; instead, in our studies we have spent time trying to make our identities as translator/interpreter and researcher visible which have highlighted some of the tensions in asking the researcher to represent the "other" cross-culturally [8–10].

Cultural Applicability of Depression Screening Tools

There is evidence that depression is underrecognized and undertreated throughout the world, especially in primary care settings [14, 62, 63]. The WHO multicountry study demonstrated that primary care physicians in their study centers detected only half of the cases of depression [64]. Treatment seeking for depressive symptoms is relatively rare in many non-Western societies and among immigrant and ethnic minority groups in the west [14, 65–67].

Primary care research in the UK shows that although people from South Asian origin visit their general practitioner more frequently than do Whites, they are less likely to have their psychological problems (specifically depression) identified [20, 31]. This is often attributed to the fact that South Asian patients may appear with mainly somatic complaints and are less willing to express depressive symptoms. Physician recognition of mental disorder is generally low in nonindustrialized countries including South Asia [68], and improving recognition rates is a challenge because of the high patient loads, poor undergraduate training in these skills, and the stigma associated with mental illness and somatic presentations of mental disorders. There is some evidence that even in industrialized countries (e.g., the UK), general practitioners' consultations regarding mental health problems are influenced by patients' cultural beliefs and practitioners' perception [69, 70].

The way of measuring and managing depression varies among groups, and cultural meanings and practices significantly shape its course. Culture influences the experience of symptoms, the terminologies used to report those, recognition of problems, decisions about treatment seeking, doctor-patient interactions, and the practices of professionals [11]. However, variations across cultures do not necessarily reflect social or medical reality, but to an unknown extent may be consequences of methodological issues, such as differences in population sampling and methods of clinical evaluation, differences in classification, and the lack of culturally appropriate measurement instruments or problems related to culturally sensitive translation and acceptability [62]. The persistent debate around two epistemological approaches within cross-cultural psychiatry is broadly based on the use of either "etic" or "emic" instruments for the recognition and evaluation of mental health illnesses, as discussed in the previous section. A good number of research studies argue that the "Western" classifications of depression proposed by both ICD-10 and DSM-IV [71] might not be simply applicable to other cultures [16, 24, 62, 72].

Accurate measurement of mental health illnesses is necessary not only for clinical/ethical reasons but also enables comparisons between different cultures. Thus, defining concepts of depression in accordance with both a psychiatric framework and lay beliefs and taking into account social contexts and cultural perspectives that give meaning to everyday life should all be incorporated into psychiatric assessment and practice [16, 73].

The recognition of depressive symptomatology is very important and requires an appropriate depression screener to be used. The past two decades have seen a number of screening instruments being designed in developed countries (notably the USA and the UK) and by the World Health Organization. Many of these screeners have been adopted by international investigators for epidemiological investigations. It is not surprising that in developed countries (e.g., the UK), practice guidelines now advocate the routine use of screening questionnaires given the high burden of mental disorders and low recognition rates in routine clinical encounters [74].

The most commonly used instrument to measure level of depression in primary care is the Patient Health Questionnaire (PHQ-9), developed in the USA [75]. The PHQ-9 consists of nine items on a 4-point Likert-type scale. It has been shown to have good sensitivity and specificity with regard to identifying cases of depression as well as being sensitive to change over time [75–78]. The WHO-5 is also a well-validated measure of positive well-being widely used in a range of settings and has been shown to have good sensitivity to depressive symptoms or depressive affect [79–83]. However, although these instruments are appropriate for English speaking (and writing) individuals, their utility in groups with high illiteracy rates and their cultural applicability have scarcely been evaluated and compared. Recognition of this has led to the concept of cultural equivalence, which can be defined as a psychological assessment tool's acceptability or applicability, reliability, and validity with people who belong to a different cultural group from those with whom the tool was originally assessed.

Although a small amount of work has been done translating written self-report instruments designed to measure depression, to date, there has been a lack of research into validating these, especially for South Asians with diabetes [6]. Self-complete instruments are not always appropriate in populations where there is a high prevalence of illiteracy or where the main language does not have an agreed written form and is only spoken [84]. Our previous research has demonstrated the potential of a range of different modes of data collection in these ethnic groups, including audio versions of questionnaires, as well as assisted completion, depending on the type of questionnaire to be completed [8, 9, 85].

The design of the ADCAD-DS was based on an action research model. The definition of action research suggested by Rapoport [86] describes it as a research method for the solution of practical problems within a real work environment while concurrently satisfying the goals of social science by engaging in mutual collaboration with research participants within an ethical framework. This method has enabled the researchers and the study participants the time and opportunity to reflect upon, and evaluate, the findings of the research as it progresses and to make changes in the study protocol when required. At the same time, this action research remains within a participatory research framework. The study developed culturally specific methods for administering and collecting reliable and valid data on psychological morbidity in South Asian people with type 2 diabetes (specifically Mirpuri and Sylheti speakers) and established the face validity of the PHQ-9 and the WHO-5. Detailed results of this part of the study have been reported elsewhere [10].

Incorporating suggestions from focus groups, participants' modified written and audio versions of both questionnaires were developed in Bengali and Sylheti, and the Sylheti version was evaluated through consultation with a group of Sylheti-speaking individuals. After initially finding many of the terms used in the two questionnaires were difficult to understand, once they were translated and adapted the items on our new versions were perceived as more relevant and acceptable in both cultures [10].

Not only did we adapt the content of the PHQ-9 and the WHO-5, we also developed new color-coded visual analogue scales to be used for recording the participants' responses to the questions. For the PHQ-9, a color-coded visual analogue scale was developed in blue, with the lightest shade for no symptoms ("not at all") and the darkest shade for most symptoms ("nearly every day"). For the WHO-5, the scale was developed in shades of green, with the lightest shade for the absence of positive mood ("not at all") and the darkest shade for most positive mood ("all of the time"). These scales were regarded very favorably by our participants, and they reported that they were much easier to complete compared to the original scales. Furthermore, using an audio recording of the questionnaires alongside the color-coded scale was perceived to be the most acceptable method of completion by the Sylheti participants [10].

Both the PHQ-9 and the WHO-5 were seen to be relevant and acceptable to the study participants, once they were translated into Mirpuri or Sylheti. Furthermore, our findings suggested that a "positive" rather than a "negative" scale could be more appropriate or more acceptable to some individuals, the WHO-5 well-being scale being one such measure [77, 79].

Our Bangladesh study was fundamentally based upon our research in the UK and the need to further validate and conduct psychometric testing of the audio versions of the PHQ-9 and WHO-5 for wider use among minority ethnic populations. We tested out both questionnaires with a bigger sample ($n=417$) of Bengali ($n=228$) and Sylheti ($n=189$) speakers in Bangladesh to further validate cultural applicability of these newly developed tools (Table 4.3). The Bangladesh study used both quantitative (a prevalence survey) and qualitative (one-to-one structured interviews for validation of instruments) data collection techniques. As illustrated in Table 4.3, our preliminary results confirmed the findings of our previous research in the UK [10] and suggest that both the Bengali and Sylheti versions of the PHQ-9 and WHO-5 are found to be similarly easy in terms of administration and completion.

The prevalence of depressive symptoms as measured by the PHQ-9 and the WHO-5 was similar regardless of the language of the questionnaires (Sylheti vs. Bengali) and method used (the standard assisted vs. independent audio). In terms of item equivalence, our findings suggest that the questions on the PHQ-9 and WHO-5 were relevant, easily understandable, and acceptable to the study participants. Most of the participants (70%) preferred the audio versions of the questionnaires. We have concluded that both the Sylheti and Bengali versions of the PHQ-9 and WHO-5 questionnaires in audio delivery format perform well and have acceptable psychometric properties for depression screening among population with high illiteracy rates, indicating cultural applicability and validity of these screeners.

Our experiences with the ADCAD-DS in the UK, as well as our work in Bangladesh, have generated ideas of translating cultural concepts across languages and understanding the languages "tied to local realities." The ADCAD-DS developed culturally equivalent content for both the PHQ-9 and the WHO-5 questionnaires in both Sylheti and Mirpuri languages and established the face validity of both questionnaires for Sylheti and Mirpuri speakers in an audio delivery format. The Bangladesh study confirmed the cultural applicability and validity of both Sylheti and Bengali versions of the PHQ-9 and WHO-5 questionnaires in audio delivery format in a population where illiteracy levels are high. The evaluation of the cultural equivalence of our assessment tools used both qualitative and quantitative measures.

Table 4.3 Summary: Bangladesh study

This study was based upon our previous research with Sylheti-speaking individuals with diabetes, living in Birmingham, UK
Our aim was to further validate and conduct psychometric testing of the audio versions of the PHQ-9 and WHO-5 for use in individuals with type 2 diabetes living in Bangladesh
Participants were recruited via three diabetes outpatient clinics in Dhaka and Sylhet. Both quantitative (a prevalence survey of depression) and qualitative (one-to-one structured interviews for validation of instruments) data collection techniques were used
We tested out two different modes of questionnaire completion: standard assisted method (with the researcher reading out the questions and the participant responding) and independent audio method (where the participant listened to the questions using an audio recorder and headphones and responded to the questions using a color-coded response sheet)
A total of 417 individuals participated in the research
High levels of undiagnosed depression and poor well-being were found among the sample overall
The prevalence of depressive symptoms as measured by the PHQ-9 and the WHO-5 was similar regardless of the method used
In both Bengali and Sylheti groups, both the PHQ-9 and the WHO-5 were found to be similarly easy to complete. However, the audio method of completion was reported as being the more acceptable method of questionnaire administration
The questions used on the PHQ-9 and WHO-5 were found to be relevant, easily understandable, and acceptable to the study participants
Audio versions of both the PHQ-9 and WHO-5 were found to be effective, valid, and culturally applicable tools for depression screening among population where illiteracy levels are high

At this point in our research, we would argue that the experience of depression is recognizable across different cultures, although researchers agree that clinical presentation may vary significantly and that mobility, migration, and globalization are likely to influence both idioms of distress and pathways to mental health care [16]. As somatic symptoms are a prominent feature of depression, existing measures of depressive symptomatology may not be appropriate for certain language groups, and it is important to adapt these according to cultural reality of the study settings and participants in order to identify those in need of psychological care and treatment.

Conclusions

This chapter demonstrates the relevance of the culture-centered approach to our understanding of mental health illness and has outlined some of the key issues related to the development of culturally sensitive depression screening tools to be used in South Asians. Awareness of culturally appropriate terminology for depression is a useful way of bridging the gap between lay and biomedical models of illness and may help improve levels of recognition, measurement, and treatment. It is possible to develop culturally appropriate instruments for measuring depressive symptoms in South Asian people with diabetes, and the measurement of depression in an international context or in other minority ethnic groups can be undertaken using similar methods and instruments (e.g., using an audio delivery format) in different cultural settings, provided appropriate action is taken to ensure cultural applicability (that involves adequate translation, adaption of culturally appropriate local terms, and validation of the cutoff score). The audio versions of both the PHQ-9 and WHO-5 questionnaires were found to be effective, valid, and culturally acceptable tools for screening depression among population where illiteracy levels are high.

References

1. Lloyd CE, Hermanns N, Nouwen A, Pouwer F, Underwood L, Winkley K. The epidemiology of diabetes and depression. In: Katon W, Maj M, Sartorius N, editors. Depression and diabetes. London: Wiley/Blackwell; 2010.
2. Ciechanowski PS, Katon WJ, Russo JE, Hirsch IB. The relationship of depressive symptoms to symptom reporting, self-care and glucose control in diabetes. Gen Hosp Psychiatry. 2003; 25:246–52.
3. Katon WJ. Clinical and health services relationships between major depression, depressive symptoms, and general medical illness. Biol Psychiatry. 2003;54:216–26.
4. Egede LE, Nietert PJ, Zheng D. Depression and all-cause and coronary mortality among adults with and without diabetes. Diabetes Care. 2005;28:1339–45.
5. Lloyd CE, Pambianco G, Orchard TJ. Does diabetes-related distress explain the presence of depressive symptoms and/or poor self-care in individuals with type 1 diabetes? Diabet Med. 2010;27(2):234–7.
6. Stone M, Lloyd CE. Psychological consequences of diabetes. In: Khunti K, Kumar S, Brodie J, editors. Diabetes UK and South Asian Health Foundation recommendations on diabetes research priorities for British South Asians. London: Diabetes UK; 2009.
7. Bhugra D, Becker MA. Migration, cultural bereavement and cultural identity. World Psychiatry. 2005;4(1):18–24.
8. Lloyd CE, Johnson MRD, Mughal S, Sturt JA, Collins GS, Roy T, et al. Securing recruitment and obtaining informed consent in minority ethnic groups in the UK. BMC Health Serv Res. 2008;8:68.
9. Lloyd CE, Sturt J, Johnson MRD, Mughal S, Collins G, Barnett AH. Development of alternative modes of data collection in South Asians with type 2 diabetes. Diabet Med. 2008;25(4): 455–62.
10. Lloyd CE, Roy T, Begum S, Mughal S, Barnett AH. Measuring Psychological well-being in South Asians with diabetes; a qualitative investigation of the PHQ-9 and the WHO-5 as potential screening tools for measuring symptoms of depression. Diabet Med. 2011;2011. doi:10.1111/j.1464-5491.2011.03481.x.
11. Kleinman A. Culture and depression. N Engl J Med. 2004;351:951–3.
12. Kleinman A. Anthropology and psychiatry: the role of culture in cross-cultural research on illness. Br J Psychiatry. 1987;151:447–54.
13. Littlewood R. From categories to contexts: a decade of the 'new cross-cultural psychiatry'. Br J Psychiatry. 1990;156:308–27.
14. Patel V. Cultural factors and international epidemiology. Br Med Bull. 2001;57:33–45.
15. Bhui K, Bhugra D. Transcultural psychiatry: some social and epidemiological research issues. Int J Soc Psychiatry. 2001;47:1–9.

16. Bhugra D, Mastrogianni A. Globalisation and mental disorders: overview with relation to depression. Br J Psychiatry. 2004;184:10–20.
17. Aidoo M, Harpham T. The explanatory models of mental health amongst low-income women and health care practitioners in Lusaka, Zambia. Health Policy Plan. 2001;16:206–13.
18. Lynch E, Medin DL. Explanatory models of illness: a study of within-culture variation. Cogn Psychol. 2006;53:285–309.
19. Hussain N, Creed F, Tomenson B. Adverse social circumstances and depression in people of Pakistani origin in the UK. Br J Psychiatry. 1997;171:434–8.
20. Commander MJ, Sashi Dharan SP, Odell SM, Surtees PG. Access to mental health care in an inner city health district I: pathways into and within specialist psychiatric services. Br J Psychiatry. 1997;170(4):312–6.
21. Jacob KS, Bhugra D, Lloyd KR, Mann AH. Common mental disorders, explanatory models and consultation behaviour among Indian women living in the UK. J R Soc Med. 1998; 91:66–71.
22. Okpaku SO. Clinical methods in transcultural psychiatry. Washington: American Psychiatric Association; 1998.
23. Kleinman A. Rethinking psychiatry. New York: Free Press; 1988.
24. Weiss MG, Raguram R, Channabasavanna SM. Cultural dimensions of psychiatric diagnosis. A comparison of DSM-III-R and illness explanatory models in south India. Br J Psychiatry. 1995;166:353–9.
25. Lloyd K, Jacob K, Patel V. The development of the short explanatory model interview and its use among primary care attenders. London: Institute of Psychiatry; 1996.
26. Bhui K. Epidemiology and social issues. In: Bhugra D, Cochrane R, editors. Psychiatry in multicultural Britain. London: Gaskell; 2001. p. 49–74.
27. Im EO, Page R, Lin LC, Tsai H, Cheng CY. Rigor in cross-cultural nursing research. Int J Nurs Stud. 2004;41:891–9.
28. Ruiz P. Ethnicity and psychopharmacology. Washington, DC: American Psychiatric Press; 2001.
29. Miyaoka Y, Miyaoka H, Montomiya T, Kitamura S, Asai M. Impact of sociodemographic and diabetes-related characteristics on depressive state among non-insulin-dependent diabetes patients. Psychiatry Clin Neurosci. 1997;51:203–6.
30. Ali S, Stone M, Peters J, Davies M, Khunti K. The prevalence of co-morbid depression in adults with type 2 diabetes: a systematic review and meta-analysis. Diabet Med. 2006;23:1165–73.
31. Bhui K, Bhugra D, Goldberg D, Dunn G, Desai M. Cultural influences on the prevalence of common mental disorder, general practitioners' assessments and help seeking among Punjabi and English people visiting their general practitioner. Psychol Med. 2001;31:815–25.
32. Herdman M, Fox-Rushby J, Badia X. A model of equivalence in the cultural adaptation of HRQoL instruments: the universalist approach. Qual Life Res. 1998;7(4):323–35.
33. Muhammad Gadit AA, Mugford G. Prevalence of depression among households in three capital cities of Pakistan: need to revise the mental health policy. PLoS One. 2007;2:e209.
34. Vogt DS, King DW, Lynda A. Focus groups in psychological assessment: enhancing content validity by consulting members of the target population. Psychol Assess. 2004;16(3):231–43.
35. Chowdhury AK. Symptomatology of depressive disorders in Bangladesh. Bangladesh Med Res Counc Bull. 1979;5:47–59.
36. Farooq S, Gahir MS, Okyere E, Sheikh AJ, Oyebode F. Somatization: a transcultural study. J Psychosom Res. 1995;39:883–8.
37. Katon W, Walker EA. Medically unexplained symptoms in primary care. J Clin Psychiatry. 1998;59(20):15–21.
38. Simon GE, VonKorff M, Piccinelli M, Fullerton C, Ormel J. An international study of the relation between somatic symptoms and depression. N Engl J Med. 1999;341:1329–35.
39. Salim N. Cultural dimensions of depression in Bangladesh: a qualitative study in two villages of Matlab. J Health Popul Nutr. 2010;28(1):95–106.

40. Desjarlais R, Eisenberg L, Good B, Kleinman A, et al. World mental health. Problems and priorities in low-income countries. Oxford: Oxford University Press; 1995.
41. Leff JP. International variations in the diagnosis of psychiatric illness. Br J Psychiatry. 1977;131:329–38.
42. Cohen MZ, Tripp-Reimer R, Smith C, Sorofman B, Lively S. Explanatory models of diabetes: patient-practitioner variation. Soc Sci Med. 1994;38:59–66.
43. Kleinman A. Patients and healers in the context of culture: an exploration of the border land between anthropology, medicine and psychiatry. Berkeley: University of California Press; 1981. p. 443.
44. Hamdi E, Yousreya A, Abou-Saleh MT. Problems in validating endogenous depression in the Arab culture by contemporary diagnostic criteria. J Affect Disord. 1997;44:131–43.
45. Sulaiman S, Bhugra D, De Silva P. Perception of depression in a community sample in Dubai. Transcult Psychiatry. 2001;38:201–18.
46. Manson SM. Culture and major depression. Current challenges in the diagnosis of mood disorders. Psychiatr Clin North Am. 1995;18:487–501.
47. Lee S. Estranged bodies, simulated harmony and misplaced cultures: neurasthenia in contemporary Chinese society. Psychosom Med. 1998;60:448–57.
48. Temple B, Young A. Qualitative research and translation dilemmas. Qual Res. 2004; 4(2):161–78.
49. Vyas A, Haidery AZ, Wiles PG, Gill S, Roberts C, Cruickshank JK. A pilot randomized trial in primary care to investigate and improve knowledge, awareness and self-management among South Asians with diabetes in Manchester. Diabet Med. 2003;20:1022–6.
50. Ansari WE. Community development and professional education in South Africa. In: Mitchell S, editor. Effective educational partnerships: experts, advocates, and scouts. Westport: Praeger; 2002. p. 217–36.
51. Bandesha G, Litva A. Perceptions of community participation and health gain in a community project for the South Asian population: a qualitative study. J Public Health. 2005;27:241–5.
52. Johnson MRD. Engaging communities and users: health and social care research with ethnic minority communities. In: Nazroo JY, editor. Health and social research in multi-ethnic societies. London: Routledge; 2006. p. 48–64.
53. Bowden A, Fox-Rushby JA. A systematic and critical review of the process of translation and adaptation of generic health-related quality of life measures in Africa, Asia, Eastern Europe, the Middle East, and South America. Soc Sci Med. 2003;57:1289–306.
54. Greenhalgh T, Helman C, Chowdhury AM. Health beliefs and folk models of diabetes in British Bangladeshis: a qualitative study. Br Med J. 1998;316:978–83.
55. Hunt SM. Cross-cultural comparability of quality of life measures. International symposium on quality of life and health. Berlin: Blackwell Verlag; 1994. p. 25–7.
56. Hunt SM, Bhopal R. Self report in clinical and epidemiological studies with non-English speakers: the challenge of language and culture. J Epidemiol Community Health. 2003; 58:618–22.
57. Simon S. Gender in translation: cultural identity and the politics of transmission. London: Routledge; 1996.
58. Young A, Ackerman J. Reflections on validity and epistemology in a study of working relations between deaf and hearing professional. Qual Health Res. 2001;11(2):179–89.
59. Ladd P. Understanding deaf culture. Clevedon: Multilingual Matters; 2003.
60. Twine F. Racial ideologies and racial methodologies. In: Twine F, Warren J, editors. Racing research researching race: methodological dilemmas in critical race studies. New York and London: New York University Press; 2000.
61. Young A. Conceptualizing parents' sign language use in bilingual early intervention. J Deaf Stud Deaf Educ. 1997;2(4):264–76.
62. Ballenger JC, Davidson JR, Lecrubier Y, Nutt DJ, Kirmayer LJ, Lépine JP, et al. Consensus statement on transcultural issues in depression and anxiety from the International Consensus Group on Depression and Anxiety. J Clin Psychiatry. 2001;62(13):47–55.

63. Lecrubier Y. Prescribing patterns for depression and anxiety worldwide. J Clin Psychiatry. 2001;62(13):31–6.
64. Sartorius N, Ustun TB, Lecrubier Y, Wittchen HU. Depression comorbid with anxiety: results from the WHO Study on Psychological Disorders in Primary Health Care. Br J Psychiatry. 1996;168(30):38–43.
65. Teja JS, Narang RL, Agarwal AK. Depression across cultures. Br J Psychiatry. 1971;119:253–60.
66. Sue S, Nakamura Y, Chung R, Yee-Bradbury C. Mental health research on Asian Americans. J Community Psychol. 1994;22:61–7.
67. Swartz MS, Wagner HR, Swanson JW, Burns BJ, George LK, Padgett DK. Administrative update: utilization of services. I. Comparing use of public and private mental health services: the enduring barriers of race and age. Community Ment Health J. 1994;34:133–44.
68. Patel V, Pereira J, Coutinho L, Fernandes R, Fernandes J, Mann A. Poverty, psychological disorder and disability in primary care attenders in Goa, India. Br J Psychiatry. 1998;171:533–6.
69. Helman C. Culture health and illness. London: Butterworth Heinemann; 1999.
70. Bhui K, Bhugra D, Goldberg D. Causal explanations of distress and general practitioners' assessments of common mental disorder among Punjabi and English attendees. Soc Psychiatry Psychiatr Epidemiol. 2002;37:38–45.
71. American Psychiatric Association. Diagnostic and statistical manual of mental disorders (DSM-IV). 4th ed. Washington, DC: APA; 1994.
72. Kirmayer LJ. Cultural variations in the clinical presentation of depression and anxiety: implications for diagnosis and treatment. J Clin Psychiatry. 2001;62(13):22–8.
73. Bhui K. Common mental disorders among people with origins in or immigrant from India and Pakistan. Int Rev Psychiatry. 1999;11:136–44.
74. NICE. Depression: management of depression in primary and secondary care. Clinical guideline. London: National Institute of Clinical Excellence, UK (NICE); 2004.
75. Spitzer RL, Kroenke K, Williams JB, Patient Health Questionnaire Primary Care Study Group. Validation and utility of a self-report version of the PRIME-MD: the PHQ primary care study. JAMA. 1999;282:1737–44.
76. Lowe B, Kroenke K, Herzog W, Grafe K. Measuring depression outcome with a brief self-report instrument: sensitivity to change of the PHQ-9. J Affect Disord. 2003;81:61–6.
77. Henkel V, Mergl R, Kohnen R, Allgaier AK, Moller HJ, Hegerl U. Use of brief depression screening tools in primary care: consideration of heterogeneity in performance in different patient groups. Gen Hosp Psychiatry. 2004;26:190–8.
78. Roy T, Lloyd CE, Pouwer F, Holt RIG, Sartorius N. Screening tools used for measuring depression among people with type 1 and type 2 diabetes: a systematic review. Diabet Med. 2011. doi:10.1111/j.1464–5491.2011.03401.x.
79. Newnham EA, Hooke GR, Page AC. Monitoring treatment response and outcomes using the World Health Organization's wellbeing index in psychiatric care. J Affect Disord. 2010;122(1–2):133–8.
80. Pouwer F, Geelhoed-Duijvestijn PH, Tack CJ, Bazelmans E, Beekman AJ, Heine RJ, et al. Prevalence of comorbid depression is high in out-patients with type 1 or type 2 diabetes mellitus. Results from three out-patient clinics in the Netherlands. Diabet Med. 2010;27(2):217–24.
81. Bech P, Olsen LR, Kjoller M, Rasmussen NK. Measuring well-being rather than absence of distress symptoms: a comparison of the SF-36 mental health subscale and the WHO-five well-being scale. Int J Methods Psychiatr Res. 2003;12:85–91.
82. Lowe B, Spitzer RL, Grafe K, Kroenke K, Quenter A, Zipfel S, et al. Comparative validity of three screening questionnaires for DSM-IV depressive disorders and physicians' diagnoses. J Affect Disord. 2004;78:131–40.
83. Awata S, Bech P, Yoshida S, Hirai M, Suzuki S, Yamashita M, et al. Reliability and validity of the Japanese version of the World Health Organization-five well-being index in the context of detecting depression in diabetic patients. Psychiatry Clin Neurosci. 2007;61:112–9.

84. Williams R, Eley S, Hunt K, Bhatt S. Has psychological distress among UK South Asians been underestimated? A comparison of three measures in the west of Scotland population. Ethn Health. 1999;2:21–9.
85. Roy T, Lloyd CE. The development of audio methods of data collection in Bangladesh. Divers Health Soc Care. 2008;5:187–98.
86. Rapoport RN. Three dilemmas in action research, with special reference to the Tavistock experience. Hum Relations. 1970;23(6):499–513.

Chapter 5
Top Ten Screening Tools for Measuring Depression in People with Diabetes

Cathy E. Lloyd and Tapash Roy

Abstract Both research and clinical practice strongly suggest that it is important to screen for and treat symptoms of depression in order to optimize diabetes self-care and facilitate both physical and psychological well-being in people with diabetes. Current evidence indicates that at least one third of people with diabetes may suffer from clinically relevant depressive disorders, with an even greater proportion reporting lower levels of symptoms that may still have a negative impact on quality of life. However, questions still remain as to the most appropriate ways of identifying people suffering from depression. Most people with diabetes are cared for by their primary care physician, and it is in this setting that there are key opportunities for screening and providing care for mental health problems.

Keywords Screening tools • Questionnaires • Depression • Diabetes • Well-being Symptomatology • Risk factors • Sensitivity • Specificity

Introduction

Both research and clinical practice strongly suggest that it is important to screen for and treat symptoms of depression in order to optimize diabetes self-care and facilitate both physical and psychological well-being in people with diabetes [1, 2].

C.E. Lloyd, Ph.D. (✉)
Faculty of Health and Social Care, The Open University,
Buckinghamshire, UK
e-mail: cathy.lloyd@open.ac.uk

T. Roy, MBBS, M.Sc., Ph.D. (✉)
Division of Social Research in Medicines and Health, School of Pharmacy,
The University of Nottingham, Nottingham, UK
e-mail: tapash_68@hotmail.com

C.E. Lloyd et al. (eds.), *Screening for Depression and Other Psychological Problems in Diabetes*,
DOI 10.1007/978-0-85729-751-8_5,

Current evidence indicates that at least one third of people with diabetes may suffer from clinically relevant depressive disorders, with an even greater proportion reporting lower levels of symptoms that may still have a negative impact on quality of life [3–5]. However, questions still remain as to the most appropriate ways of identifying people suffering from depression. Most people with diabetes are cared for by their primary care physician, and it is in this setting that there are key opportunities for screening and providing care for mental health problems.

In this chapter, we review some of the most widely used tools available for screening for depressive symptomatology in people with diabetes. People with depression are more likely to attend their primary care facility than visit a mental health professional; however, primary care physicians have little experience in detecting depressive symptomatology which may therefore go undetected and untreated [6]. Furthermore, diagnostic interviews (considered to be the gold standard for identifying depression) are time-consuming, costly, and require training in their application. Brief screening instruments or questionnaires are quick and simple to administer, and most have been shown to approximate clinically significant levels of depressive disorder at certain cut points or scores. It should be remembered however that most screening tools are just that – they screen for symptoms of depression but are not intended for use as a diagnostic tool but as a first step towards a definitive diagnosis usually using a clinical interview. The majority of available screening tools measure the presence/absence of depression, the type of symptoms present, and also the severity of symptoms. The main limitation for most instruments is, unlike diagnostic interviews, the requirement for literacy unless one wishes to orally administer the questionnaire.

It is common practice to distinguish between "major" and "minor" depression, although this can be misleading; minor depression can be more severe and longer-lasting than major depression and can have an equally serious impact on overall health and well-being. It is also important to note that people may experience depressive symptoms that do not satisfy the criteria for a diagnosis of either major or minor depression, but nevertheless these symptoms may cause a lot of distress, impact on quality of life, and require some type of intervention or support. Routine depression screening in diabetes patients is feasible in different ways. The current risk of an individual with diabetes experiencing symptoms of depression can be assessed by the presence or absence of particular risk factors (see Table 5.1). A range of self-report screening tools have been devised for use in both research and clinical practice, many of which have been shown to measure symptoms that approximate clinical levels of depression (see Table 5.1).

Many screening instruments have been assessed according to their *sensitivity*, that is to say how well they perform in terms of identifying all the people with symptoms of depression ("true positives"), and *specificity*, which refers to the ability of a screening tool to identify people with symptoms of depression rather than other psychological morbidities.

Table 5.1 Symptoms of depression measured using self-report instruments

Feeling sad/depressed mood
Inability to sleep
Early waking
Lack of interest/enjoyment
Tiredness/lack of energy
Loss of appetite
Feelings of guilt/worthlessness
Recurrent thoughts about death/suicide

Sensitivity is defined as:

$$\frac{\text{Number of true positives (cases of depression)}}{\text{Number of true positives + number of false negatives}}$$

Specificity is defined as:

$$\frac{\text{Number of true negatives}}{\text{Number of true negatives + false positives}}$$

The screening performance of different tools is usually evaluated according to these two criteria (sensitivity and specificity). For clinical practice, the positive and negative predictive values are also of considerable interest, and these will be discussed towards the end of the chapter. Many screening tools contain both cognitive and somatic symptoms of depression, and these may overlap with some of the symptoms of diabetes, especially when glycemic control is poor or when the complications of diabetes (e.g., heart disease, diabetic retinopathy, kidney failure, peripheral neuropathy) start to develop. These symptoms include loss of/increase in appetite, difficulties in sleeping, fatigue, loss of energy, and weight loss. It may be difficult therefore to disentangle reported symptoms which may relate to depression or to diabetes or even both. This is important because it may affect clinical decision-making and treatment recommendations. However, it has been argued that by removing the somatic items from a depression scale, while helping to avoid the problem of overlap between symptoms of physical disease and psychological status, this may actually lead to underrecognition of depressive disorder [7]. The cognitive symptoms of depression may also be affected by the experience of having diabetes, for example, individuals may have a fear of the future or have feelings of hopelessness which may be related to diabetes and its complications or may have more to do with other aspects of their lives. There may also be differences in the applicability of different screening instruments in particular subgroups, for example, in older people, in men or women, and in certain cultural or ethnic minority groups. It is important to keep these issues in mind when deciding on which instrument to use.

In this chapter, we review ten of the most common tools used to measure symptoms of depression in people with diabetes; these are:

1. The Center for Epidemiological Studies Depression Scale: CES-D
2. The Beck Depression Inventory: BDI
3. The Patient Health Questionnaire: PHQ-9
4. The Hospital Anxiety and Depression Scale: HADS
5. The Zung Self-Rating Depression Scale: ZSDS
6. The Medical Outcomes Short Form (SF) 36/12
7. The Hamilton Psychiatric Rating Scale for Depression: HRSD
8. The General Health Questionnaire: GHQ-12
9. The World Health Organization Well-Being Scale: WHO-5/ WHO Major Depression Inventory: WHO MDI
10. The Montgomery/Asberg Depression Rating Scale: MADRS

The above tools are only a sample of the many tools available to screen for depression; for the purposes of this chapter, we have focused on those that have been most commonly used in people with diabetes. We have published elsewhere a more comprehensive and systematic review [8].

The Center for Epidemiological Studies Depression Scale (CES-D)

Author: L.S. Radloff

Year first used: 1977

Mode of completion: Self-complete

Country where developed: USA

Languages available: English, Spanish, Dutch, Croatian, and Chinese

The CES-D is one of the most commonly used measures to screen for symptoms of depression [9]. It consists of a 20-item self-complete scale measuring the frequency of symptoms of depression during the past week on a four-point scale, ranging from "rarely or none of the time" to "most or all of the time." Higher CES-D scores indicate greater depressive symptomatology, with scores of 16 or higher being indicative of clinically significant levels of depression, and scores of 10–15 indicating moderate levels of symptomatology [9].

One advantage of the CES-D is that it does not include many somatic items which could be confounded with the symptoms of poorly controlled diabetes, for example, tiredness or weight loss. Questions relating to symptoms such as loss of appetite and restless sleep (which may be related to symptoms of diabetes) are included however.

CES-D Sample Questions

Using the scale below, indicate the number which best describes how often you felt or behaved this way – during the past week

1 = Rarely or none of the time (less than 1 day)
2 = Some or a little of the time (1–2 days)
3 = Occasionally or a moderate amount of time (3–4 days)
4 = Most or all of the time (5–7 days)

During the past week:

- I was bothered by things that usually don't bother me
- I felt that everything I did was an effort
- I enjoyed life
- I felt sad

The CES-D has been administered in a range of different populations, in people with type 1 and type 2 diabetes as well as in nondiabetic populations, and has been found to have high sensitivity and specificity [10]. Although it has been found to have a high negative predictive value (i.e., a low rate of false positives), it has also been found to have only a moderate positive predictive value (i.e., a high rate of false positives) [10]. In one recent study comparing several depression screening tools, the CES-D was found to be the best predictor of depression in people with type 2 diabetes [11]. This study also examined the overlap of symptoms of diabetes and depression and reported that the CES-D had the best ability to discriminate between depression and other nondepressive symptoms. This is important because a number of studies (in both type 1 and type 2 diabetes) have shown a high correlation between depression symptoms, measured by the CES-D, and symptoms of diabetes-related distress [1, 2, 12, 13]. Furthermore, research suggests a strong link between the persistence of depressive symptoms over time and diabetes-related distress [14, 15]. These links have implications for clinical practice and especially treatment decisions.

Originally developed in the English language, the CES-D has been translated into a number of other languages (see above); however, there remains very little evidence as to the cultural applicability of the CES-D. Some studies have reported ethnic differences in rates of depression using the CES-D [16], but overall the findings are equivocal with other studies reporting little difference between ethnic groups [17]. One study using the CES-D showed little difference in rates of reported depressive symptomatology when comparing African Americans, Hispanics, and white Caucasians, but there were differences in treatment uptake which may reflect those cultural differences [17].

The CES-D has been used in studies investigating the relationship between depression and diabetes complications as well as other conditions including cerebrovascular disease, arthritis, and cancer [18]. For example, it has been used to examine depressive symptoms in people with chronic pain [19]. In this study, removing the somatic items did not improve the sensitivity or accuracy of the scale. A review by Wulsin et al. [20] included several studies that used the CES-D, all of which showed a positive relationship between high CES-D scores and coronary artery disease.

The CES-D has been adapted to provide two shorter formats – an 8-item and a 10-item scale – in order to improve acceptability in certain populations. As the content of these scales varies however, there is little currently known about the validity of these scales. A more complete review of the shortened CES-D can be found in Grzywacz et al. – in his evaluation of the utility of three versions of this instrument in Mexican American migrants [21].

The Beck Depression Inventory (BDI)

Author: A.T. Beck
Time of first use: 1961
Mode of completion: Self-complete
Country where developed: USA
Languages available: English, German, Chinese, Dutch, Finnish, French, Korean, Swedish, and Turkish

The BDI was originally developed in the 1960s [22, 23]; however, it has more recently been updated and renamed the BDI-II [24]. Both versions are still in use, so it is useful to mention the differences between the two measures. The original BDI consisted of 21 items, where the respondent was asked to indicate how they have been feeling during the past week. The BDI-II also consists of 21 items; however, symptoms must have occurred during the past 2 weeks – this is in line with the DSM-IV criteria. There are also a substantial number of wording changes, with most items being reworded. Some examples of these are given below.

BDI (original version)	BDI-II (updated version)
Symptoms during the past week	Symptoms during the past 2 weeks
Item 1:	Item 1:
I do not feel sad	I do not feel sad
I feel sad	I feel sad much of the time
I am so sad all the time and I can't snap out of it	I am sad all the time
I am so sad or unhappy that I can't stand it	I am so sad or unhappy that I can't stand it
Item 2:	Item 2:
I am not particularly discouraged about the future	I am not discouraged about my future

I feel discouraged about the future	I feel more discouraged about my future than I used to be
I feel I have nothing to look forward to	I do not expect things to work out for me
I feel that the future is hopeless and that things cannot improve	I feel my future is hopeless and will only get worse
Item 16:	Item 16:
I can sleep as well as usual	I have not experienced any change in my sleeping pattern
I don't sleep as well as I used to	I sleep somewhat more than usual/I sleep somewhat less than usual
I wake up 1–2 h earlier than usual and find it hard to get back to sleep	I sleep a lot more than usual/I sleep a lot less than usual
I wake up several hours earlier than I used to and cannot get back to sleep	I sleep most of the day/I wake up 1–2 h early and can't get back to sleep

The BDI-II was developed in 1996 in response to the new edition of the Diagnostic and Statistical Manual of Mental Disorders (DSM-IV) which contained a number of changes to the diagnostic criteria for major depression. The BDI-II is one of the screening tools recommended by the English government Department of Health for use in primary care but again is rarely used due to the cost implications. It is much more commonly used in research studies [8]. The cutoffs for minor and major depression on the original BDI were 10 and 16 respectively; on the BDI-II, these are 14–19 (mild), 20–28 (moderate), and 29+ (severe).

The original BDI has been shown to have high sensitivity and specificity (87% and 81% respectively) and high negative predictive value (83%) [25]. Positive predictive value has also been found to be good (66%) [25]. Both instruments contain cognitive and somatic items, which have led to questions being raised with regard to the applicability of the BDI in people with diabetes. Nevertheless, the BDI has been and continues to be used in much of the research in this area.

The BDI has been used in studies of the prevalence of depression in type 1 and type 2 diabetes [26, 27] and in studies of the development of diabetes complications [28]. In the latter study, a longitudinal prospective investigation of the development of complications in people with type 1 diabetes, raised BDI scores were associated with subsequent diagnosis of coronary artery disease [28]. The BDI-II was recently used in a study of depression comparing people with type 1 diabetes with a cohort free of this condition [29]. The authors reported an increased rate of depressive symptoms in those with diabetes as well as more antidepressant use.

The BDI-II has been validated in adults without diabetes including college students and people attending psychiatric clinics [24]. It has also been evaluated for use in detecting depression in primary care and has been found to be a valid tool in such settings [30]. Translated versions are available in a number of languages including German, Chinese, Dutch, Finnish, French, Korean, Swedish, and Turkish.

The Patient Health Questionnaire (PHQ-9)

Authors: R. Spitzer, K. Kroenke
Time of first use: 1999
Mode of completion: Self-complete
Country where developed: USA
Languages available: English, Bengali, German, Thai, Hindi, Gujarati, Punjabi, Japanese, Arabic, Spanish, Danish, Dutch, Cantonese, and many more

The PHQ-9 was devised in the USA for use in primary care and is based on the diagnostic criteria for major depressive disorder – as laid out in the Diagnostic and Statistical Manual of Mental Disorders (DSM-IV) [31, 32]. There are two aspects to this tool: a nine-item screen to assess symptoms that have occurred during the last 2 weeks, followed by the determination of a symptom severity score to make a decision as to the appropriate treatment. Scores of 10–14 on the 9-item screen are indicative of minor depression, scores of 15–19 are indicative of moderately severe depression, and scores of 20+ indicate clinically significant levels of depression. The PHQ-9 has been found to have high sensitivity (73%) and specificity (98%) [33], as well as good positive and negative predictive values.

Possibly due to its relative brevity and ease of use, the PHQ-9 has been found to be acceptable in a number of different patient groups, including people with and also without diabetes. It is easy to score and subsequently interpret. However, several items on the scale could be said to be confounded with the symptoms of diabetes, for example, tiredness, lack of energy, and poor appetite/overeating. The PHQ-9 is one of three screening instruments recommended by the English Department of Health for use in primary care. It has begun to be used more extensively in research settings, for example, in the Pathways Study [33]. This latter study used the PHQ-9 to screen for depression in over 4,000 individuals with diabetes. Significant correlates of depression included treatment with insulin, poorer glycemic control, smoking, high body mass index, and the presence of diabetes complications. The Pathways Study researchers have also reported a link between major depression and poor self-care, including low levels of physical activity, unhealthy diet, and less concordance with diabetes medications [33].

The Patient Health Questionnaire (PHQ-9)
Sample questions:
Over the last 2 weeks how often have you been bothered by any of the following problems?
(Not at all/several days/more than half the days/nearly every day)

- Little interest or pleasure in doing things
- Feeling down, depressed, or hopeless
- Trouble falling or staying asleep
- Feeling tired or having little energy
- Poor appetite or overeating

Henkel et al. [6] compared the PHQ-9 with two other instruments and found it had the highest specificity and positive predictive value. The authors also reported that it was the most powerful screening instrument for major depression probably because it was developed according to the DSM-IV criteria for major depressive disorder. It has been reported recently that the PHQ-9 is able to detect depression outcome and is sensitive to change over time [34].

The PHQ-9 has been used in longitudinal studies of individuals with diabetes to investigate the role of depression in the development of cardiovascular disease as well as other diabetes complications [35]. A recent study showed a high correlation between the PHQ-9 and frequency of reported diabetes symptoms such as cold hands and feet, numb hands and feet, polyuria, excessive hunger, abnormal thirst, shakiness, blurred vision, feeling faint, and feeling sleepy [36]. The authors argue for the importance of treating depression irrespective of whether the symptoms of depression are a cause or consequence of the diabetes symptoms.

There are versions of the PHQ-9 in more than 45 languages; however, as with many other screening tools, the cultural applicability of this instrument has not, to date, been fully tested. A recent study in India adapted the PHQ-9 to suit local conditions [37]. The adapted version consisted of 12 (rather than 9) items as three items were divided into two. Response options were also modified – from a 4-point scale to a yes/no response as this was deemed easier to use. The study found the new version of the PHQ to be a valid and reliable instrument for screening for depression in India.

A study in the UK has just been completed which has developed audio versions of the PHQ-9 for use in Bangladeshi patients who speak Sylheti and Pakistani patients who speak Mirpuri [38]. Neither Sylheti nor Mirpuri has an agreed written form, and there are high levels of illiteracy in these populations, so an audio format is more suited to their needs. This research has shown a high acceptability of the audio questionnaires, in spite of the often-perceived stigma associated with poor mental health and subsequent reluctance to discuss or admit to feeling depressed. However, further work still needs to be done in order to validate these new tools in a larger population.

The Hospital Anxiety and Depression Scale (HADS)

Authors: R.P. Snaith, A.S. Zigmond

Time of first use: 1983

Mode of completion: Self-complete

Country where developed:

Languages available: UK, French, Swedish, Italian, Portuguese, Spanish, Arabic, Urdu, German, Greek, Dutch, and Persian

The HADS is a brief self-complete scale measuring the presence of symptoms of anxiety (7 items) and depression (7 items) during the past week [39]. It has been used extensively with people with long-term physical health problems, including diabetes [40–42], and its utility and acceptability in people with diabetes as well as other long-term conditions have been well demonstrated [40, 43]. It is also one of the screening tools recommended by the English Department of Health for use in primary care; however, it is rarely used due to the financial cost involved. The HADS does not include somatic items which could be confounded with the symptoms of poorly controlled diabetes. Scores on the depression scale between 8 and 10 are considered to approximate mild symptomatology, scores between 11 and 14 indicate moderate symptoms, and scores of 15 or higher indicate severe depressive symptomatology.

Some data on specificity and sensitivity are available, with one review of existing studies estimating an average sensitivity and specificity of around 80% [44]. Positive and negative predictive values were not calculated in this case for reasons of appropriateness due to their sensitivity to the varying prevalence of "true cases" of depression observed in the different studies. This report also found that the HADS performed well in assessing the severity of symptoms in a range of patient populations including those already identified as having physical health problems as well as those without. In a recent study in Ireland, the prevalence of symptoms of both anxiety and depression was found to be higher in people with diabetes compared to general population samples [45]. The same study also observed higher rates of depression in those with diabetes complications, a finding supported in other studies [41].

The HADS has been used in research where other long-term physical health conditions have been the focus, including coronary artery disease [46], cancer [43, 47], and chronic pain [48, 49]. Research has also been conducted in people with diabetes and neuropathy and has found increased HADS scores associated with reports of greater neuropathic pain [50, 51].

Hospital Anxiety and Depression Scale (HADS)
Sample questions:
Read each item below and underline the reply which is closest to how you have been feeling in the past week
Depression:
I can laugh at the funny side of things

- As much as I always could
- Not quite so much now
- Definitely not so much now
- Not at all

I feel cheerful

- Never
- Not often
- Sometimes
- Most of the time

Anxiety
I feel tense or "wound up"

- Most of the time
- A lot of the time
- From time to time, occasionally
- Not at all

I get a sort of frightened feeling like "butterflies" in the stomach

- Not at all
- Occasionally
- Quite often
- Very often

Research indicates that the HADS, while originally designed for people with physical illness attending a medical setting, is also a valid tool for use in community settings [39]. It has also been found to be sensitive to change both during the course of a physical illness and in response to intervention [52].

The HADS is available in most European languages (e.g., French, German, Dutch, Italian, Portuguese, Spanish, Greek) as well as Arabic, Urdu, and Persian [43, 44, 53]. The Persian version has been shown to be an acceptable, reliable, and valid measure of psychological distress among Iranian cancer patients [43]. Although the HADS has been translated widely, the cultural applicability of this instrument has not yet been specifically addressed. Furthermore, there is some (largely anecdotal) evidence that the cultural equivalency of the severity scale itself may be questioned and may not translate easily into different levels/intensity of symptoms (Ali, 2010, personal communication). This can be said for a number of the scales considered here; it is not only an important consideration for the HADS.

Zung Self-Rating Depression Scale (ZSDS)

Author: W.W.K Zung

Time of first use: 1965

Mode of completion: Self-complete

Country where developed: USA

Available languages: English, Chinese, Finnish, Japanese, Russian, Italian, and Greek

The Zung Self-Rating Depression Scale (ZSDS), developed in the 1960s, is a 20-item scale designed for self-completion, with respondents asked to indicate how they feel on a 4-point scale for each item [54]. The maximum score available is 80, with scores between 50 and 69 indicating depression and with scores of 70 or higher suggesting severe depression.

Zung Self-Rating Depression Scale (ZSDS)
Example items:
Please read each statement and decide how much of the time the statement describes how you've been feeling during the past 2 weeks:
(A little of the time/some of the time/good part of the time/most of the time)

- I feel downhearted and blue
- I get tired for no reason
- I feel hopeful about the future
- I still enjoy the things I used to
- I have trouble sleeping at night

The Zung scale does contain some somatic items – for example, sleep disturbance and weight loss – which may be confounded with the symptoms of diabetes. However, this scale has been shown to have good validity and internal consistency in the general population [55], and it has been used successfully in a number of studies in people with diabetes. Indeed, the ZSDS has also been shown to have good sensitivity (100%) and modest specificity (59%) for detecting major depression in people with diabetes when using Zung scores of 40 or more [56]. It has been stressed, however, that higher scores on the ZSDS are only an indicator of clinically significant depressive symptoms, not a diagnosis of depressive disorder. In a study in China, Xu and colleagues found increased rates of depression (defined as scores of 40 or greater on the ZSDS) in women with diabetes, in those with longer durations of diabetes, and in those with a greater number of diabetes complications [57]. The proportion of people with diabetes reporting depressive symptoms was similar to that reported in Western countries. Furthermore, glycemic control was significantly poorer in those with higher depression scores. Other studies in China [58, 59] have also used the ZSDS and found similar rates of depressive symptoms in people with both ongoing and newly diagnosed diabetes. An earlier study, which was conducted in Finland [60], used a cutoff of 45 to indicate clinically significant levels of depressive symptoms on the ZSDS and found higher rates of depression in people with diagnosed compared to undiagnosed diabetes. A prospective study in Japanese men who were followed up for 8 years after completing the ZSDS found that those who had moderate or severe levels of depressive symptoms (scores ≥48 on the ZSDS) were 2.3 times more likely to develop type 2 diabetes compared to those with lower scores [61].

Recently, Zung developed a second scale designed to serve as an adjunct to the ZSDS in order to obtain an interviewer rating of the severity and symptoms of depression in line with diagnostic criteria [62]. Zung has suggested that the combination of the self-report screen and the clinical interview can work together to help more easily identify those in need of treatment for depressive disorder.

Zung Depression Status Inventory (DSI)	
Signs/symptoms of depression	Interview questions (responses: none, mild, moderate, or severe)
Depressed mood	Do you ever feel sad or depressed?
Fatigue	How easily do you get tired?
Hopelessness	How hopeful do you feel about the future?

To our knowledge, data on the use of the DSI in people with diabetes has not been reported, and we have found only four studies which reported using the DSI in nondiabetic populations. In one of those [63], depression status was associated with poorer working conditions such as isolation. The DSI has been used successfully in two studies in older people [64, 65] and has also been used in a randomized controlled trial for treatment of depression [66].

The Medical Outcomes Study Short Form 36 (SF-36) [and the Short Form 12]

Author: JE Ware
Time of first use: 1988
Mode of completion: Self-complete
Country where developed: USA
Available languages: English, Spanish, Hawaiian, Croatian, and Japanese
The Medical Outcomes Study (MOS) SF-36 was developed as a tool for measuring general population patient outcomes in different domains, both physical and mental health as well as a more general assessment of well-being [67]. There are eight separate outcomes or concepts addressed in the SF-36, and there are manuals with population norms given to support the interpretation of data.

The Medical Outcomes Study Short Form 36 (SF-36)
Eight domains:

1. Physical functioning: limitations in performing physical activities due to health
2. Role limitation – physical: problems with work/other daily activities due to physical health
3. Bodily pain: reported pain or limitations due to pain
4. Role limitation – emotional: problems with work/other daily activities due to emotional problems
5. General health: evaluation of personal health and whether it might deteriorate

6. Vitality: evaluation of personal energy levels
7. Social functioning: extent to which normal social activities can be performed without interference from physical/emotional problems
8. Mental health: extent to which feelings of nervousness or depression are experienced

The mental health subscale consists of five items and includes anxiety, depression, loss of behavioral/emotional control, and psychological well-being. An overall mental health summary score can also be derived by collating the scores from 4 of the SF-36 domains including the mental health domain along with the role limitation – emotional, social functioning, and vitality components.

The Mental Health Dimension of the SF-36

How much of the time during the past month:

- Have you been a very nervous person?
- Have you felt so down in the dumps that nothing could cheer you up?
- Have you felt calm and peaceful?
- Have you felt downhearted and blue?
- Have you been a happy person?

The SF-36 is referred to as a "generic measure" of health-related quality of life because it measures well-being in a way that is relevant to all people rather than just those with a particular condition. However, it has been used in a number of studies in people with diabetes as well as in studies of the general population. For example, in the Whitehall study of British civil servants [68], mental health, as measured by the five items on the SF-36, improved with age but was poorer in women and in those working in lower-grade jobs. In a general population household survey in Australia, the combination of diabetes and depression was associated with poorer scores on all 8 dimensions of the SF-36 but had the strongest impact on overall physical health [69]. A study of people with diabetes [70], where only the mental health subscale of the SF-36 was used, found that poorer mental health was significantly associated with lower perceived general health and also poorer perceived diabetes control (although not with actual levels of glycemic control). The SF-36 has also been used to measure change in health-related quality of life, as for example, in a study by Claiborne and Massaro [71]. This study involved assessing patients with type 2 diabetes prior to and after receiving diabetes education over a 6-month period. Mental health summary scores decreased significantly over time and were associated with greater risk for depressive disorder; however, physical functioning remained the same. Clinically significant levels of depressive symptoms have been found to be associated with poorer SF-36 scores in other studies in people with diabetes [56].

Although the SF-36 is still used extensively, a shorter questionnaire, the SF-12, has been developed [72]. The SF-12 contains the same 8 dimensions as the SF-36 which can be used to examine the separate components of health-related quality of life as before, along with the two summary scores for physical and mental health. A detailed explanation for the development of the SF-12 and a comparison of the two instruments are available from the authors [73]. Recent research using the SF-12 reported associations between poorer SF-12 scores and pain severity in people with type 2 diabetes [74].

Hamilton Depression Rating Scale (HDRS)

Author(s): M. Hamilton
Time of first use: 1960
Self/expert/nonexpert complete: Expert
Country where developed: USA
Languages available in: English, German, Thai, French, Polish, Italian, and Turkish

The Hamilton Depression Rating Scale (HDRS) was designed in 1960 as a psychiatric tool to measure severity of depressive symptoms rather than the presence or absence of depression [75]. There are a number of different versions, but the one most commonly used is the 17-item questionnaire. Unlike most screening tools, the HDRS should be used by health care professionals or trained interviewers rather than completed by the individual patient [76].

The HDRS is commonly used in medical research, including studies in people with diabetes [77, 78] as well as other long-term conditions such as cancer [79]. It was at one time considered to be the gold standard for measuring severity of depressive symptoms, but there have been some criticisms of the scale in recent years particularly because of the overlap between the somatic symptoms of depression and those of physical ill-health which may impact on sensitivity [80]. To some extent this may be because it has been used inappropriately in nondepressed populations, whereas it is designed only for use in individuals who have already been identified as depressed.

Hamilton Depression Rating Scale (HDRS)
Sample questions from the 17-item HDRS:
(Complete the scale based on a structured interview)
Depressed mood

0 Absent
1 These feeling states indicated only on questioning
2 These feeling states spontaneously reported verbally

3 Communicates these feeling states nonverbally, i.e., through facial expression, posture, voice, and tendency to weep
4 Patient reports virtually only these feeling states in his/her spontaneous verbal and nonverbal communication

Insomnia: middle of the night

0 No difficulty
1 Patient complains of being restless and disturbed during the night
2 Waking during the night – any getting out of bed rates 2 (except for purpose of voiding)

Anxiety somatic (physiological concomitants of anxiety) such as:

Gastrointestinal – dry mouth, wind, indigestion, diarrhea, cramps, belching
Cardiovascular – palpitations, headaches
Respiratory – hyperventilation, sighing
Urinary frequency
Sweating
0 Absent
1 Mild
2 Moderate
3 Severe
4 Incapacitating

Respondents are asked to indicate the presence and severity of depressive symptoms during the past week on a 3- or 5-point scale, depending on the item being considered. A score of 0–6 is regarded as indicating the absence of depression, scores of 7–17 as mild levels of symptomatology, scores between 8 and 24 as moderate depression, and scores greater than 24 as indicative of severe levels of depression. The HDRS has been shown to correlate highly with the BDI and a number of other scales.

The HDRS has been translated in to a number of other languages, including German, Thai, French, Polish, Italian, and Turkish; however, the cultural validity of these translations is not known.

The General Health Questionnaire (GHQ)

Author(s): D. Goldberg, P. Williams
Time of first use: 1988
Self/expert/nonexpert complete: Self-complete
Country where developed: UK
Languages available in: English, German, Italian, Spanish, Czech, Iranian, and more

The GHQ was originally developed by David Goldberg and Paul Williams, and there are now four versions of this instrument: the GHQ-28, GHQ-30, GHQ-60, and the GHQ-12, the latter being the tool most commonly used in research (see http://www.gl-assessment.co.uk/health_and_psychology/resources/general_health_questionnaire/faqs.asp?css=1). There are some financial costs involved, and a number of translations are available via MAPI (see trust@mapi.fr).

The GHQ-12 can be scored according to the original method (0 – 0 – 1 – 1) or using a Likert-type score (0 – 1 – 2 – 3) which has been thought to be more useful

General Health Questionnaire (GHQ-12)
Sample questions:
We want to know how your health has been in general over the last few weeks
(Better than usual/same as usual/less than usual/much less than usual)
Have you recently:

Been able to concentrate on what you're doing?
Lost much sleep over worry?
Felt you couldn't overcome your difficulties?
Been feeling unhappy or depressed?
Been losing confidence in yourself?
Been thinking of yourself as a worthless person?

when assessing the severity of depressive symptoms. It has been shown to have high sensitivity and specificity and works as well as the longer instrument (the GHQ-28) in detecting cases of depression [81]. The GHQ-12 has been found to be a valid instrument in countries such as India, Brazil, China, and Greece [81]. It has also been shown to have high sensitivity and specificity when used in South Asian migrants living in the UK [82, 83]. Only a small number of studies have been conducted in people with diabetes; however, studies in people with diabetes in Spain and Finland, using the GHQ-12, have illustrated its utility in evaluating mental health status in this group [84, 85].

The Well-Being Index: WHO-5 and the WHO Major Depression Inventory: WHO-MDI

Authors: P. Bech/WHO Collaborating Centre for Mental Health, Denmark
Time of first use: 1993
Self/expert/nonexpert complete: self/expert
Country where developed: Denmark
Languages available in: English, Danish, Spanish, French, German, Russian, Farsi, Urdu, and Bengali

The Well-Being Index, or WHO-5 as it became known, was developed in the 1990s as a derivation of a larger (28-item) scale designed to measure quality of life in people with diabetes [86–88]. Although the title of the scale suggests it was developed by the World Health Organization, this is not exactly the case, but it was first used by the WHO Collaborating Centre for Mental Health in Denmark. Interestingly, there are two items on the WHO-5 which may possibly be associated with symptoms of poorly controlled diabetes (feeling active and vigorous, waking up feeling fresh and rested). This scale is unusual because it is a positive mood scale, measuring the absence rather than the presence of negative mood during the past 2 weeks. Scores below 13 indicate poor well-being and indicate the need for further investigation for depression.

Although this scale measures a broader spectrum of emotional well-being, sensitivity and specificity with regard to identifying cases of depression have been shown to be high (100% and 78% respectively) [25]. In the same study, positive predictive value was below average (45%) but negative predictive value excellent (100%).

Well-Being Index: WHO-5

Please indicate for each of the five statements which is closest to how you have been feeling over the last 2 weeks
(All of the time/most of the time/more than half of the time/less than half of the time/some of the time/at no time)

I have felt cheerful and in good spirits
I have felt calm and relaxed
I have felt active and vigorous
I woke up feeling fresh and rested
My daily life has been filled with things that interest me

http://www.who-5.org/

The WHO-5 has been used effectively in a study of the prevalence of depression in individuals with type 2 diabetes, in both people from white European and South Asian backgrounds [89]. It has also been validated in a Japanese sample of people with diabetes [90]. A recent study reported that higher (i.e., better) WHO-5 scores were associated with adequate glycemic control [91]. In the same study, poorer WHO-5 scores were associated with reports of neuropathic pain.

This tool has been translated into many other languages including Danish, Spanish, French, German, Russian, and Urdu. Although the cultural applicability of this short screen has yet to be fully clarified, there is evidence of the WHO-5 having good reliability and validity in languages other than English [92, 93].

The WHO-5 has been used in studies in community or primary care populations as well as in research in people with long-term conditions other than diabetes, for example, cancer and heart disease [94]. In a comparison of the PHQ-9, GHQ-12, and the WHO-5 in a primary care sample, the latter demonstrated superior sensitivity and false negative rate [6]. This study also suggested that the WHO-5 had greater diagnostic ability compared to the other tools. In our own research in South Asians with type 2 diabetes, the WHO-5 was preferred to the PHQ-9 because it was a positive rather than negative scale; however, some respondents were critical of the scale on which their responses could be made, finding it difficult to translate [38]. Careful work still needs to be done in order to ensure the cultural relevance of this scale, as with other screening tools, before we can be sure that we are actually measuring depressive symptomatology in minority ethnic groups.

Major Depression Inventory: MDI

The MDI is a 10-item screening tool for use in primary care to screen for major depression, based on the ICD-10 criteria. It is recommended that the MDI is used in those individuals who score poorly on the WHO-5 positive well-being scale (http://www.cure4you.dk/354/The_Depcare_Project.pdf). Scoring of the questionnaire and diagnosis of depression are dependent on a series of algorithms which match ICD-10 or DSM-IV criteria. The MDI can also be used to measure the severity of depression, with a range of 0 (no depression) to 50 (severe depression). The MDI is reported to have high sensitivity (86%) and specificity (86%) [95]. Similarly, sensitivity and specificity with regard to identifying major depression have been shown to be high with the Greek translation of the MDI (0.86% and 0.94% respectively) [96]. When used in a sample of patients with different states of depression, the Spanish version of MDI has also been found to have an adequate internal and external validity [97]. There are several items on the scale which could be confounded with the symptoms of diabetes, such as trouble sleeping at night and decreases/increases in appetite.

WHO Major Depression Inventory: WHO MDI

Sample questions:

The following questions ask about how you have been feeling over the last 2 weeks (All the time/most of the time/slightly more than half the time/slightly less than half of the time/some of the time/at no time)

- Have you felt low in spirits or sad?
- Have you lost interest in your daily activities?
- Have you felt lacking in energy and strength?
- Have you felt that life wasn't worth living?
- Have you suffered from reduced appetite?

http://www.who-5.org/

The MDI is available in a number of languages including English, French, Danish, Dutch, German, Spanish, Finnish, Swedish, Serbian, and Turkish. Although we have not found any research in people with diabetes, it has been successfully used in studies in the community and in primary care populations in people with long-term conditions, for example, chronic pain and Parkinson's disease [98, 99].

Montgomery/Asberg Depression Rating Scale: MADRS

Author(s): S.A. Montgomery and M. Asberg
Time of first use: 1979
Self/expert/nonexpert complete: Expert
Country where developed: UK/Sweden
Languages available in: English, Swedish, Bengali, and Urdu

This scale was developed to be used in pharmacological studies, where the sensitivity and accuracy of measuring change in symptoms over time were of key importance [100]. It was developed in both English and Swedish and consisted of ten items. It was designed to be completed by a trained health care professional during an interview rather than to be self-completed. There are a number of studies which have demonstrated its utility in research evaluating the efficacy of treatments for depression, and it has been shown to be sensitive to change [101].

Montgomery Asberg Depression Rating Scale: MADRS
Sample questions (how you have been feeling during the past 3 days)
Reported sadness (rate according to intensity, duration, and the extent to which the mood is reported to be influenced by events)

0 Occasional sadness in keeping with the circumstances
1
2 Sad or low but brightens up without difficulty
3
4 Pervasive feelings of sadness or gloominess. The mood is still influenced by external circumstances
5
6 Continuous or unvarying sadness, misery, or despondency

Reduced sleep (representing the experience of reduced duration or depth of sleep compared to the subject's own normal pattern when well)

0 Sleeps as usual
1
2 Slight difficulty dropping off to sleep or slightly reduced, light, or fitful sleep
3
4 Sleep reduced or broken by at least 2 h

5
6 Less than 2 or 3 h sleep

SA Montgomery and M Asberg, 1979

The Self-Report MADRS

A brief 9-item self-report version of this scale, the MADRS-S, has also been developed [102]. This scale consists of similar items assessing patients' mood, feelings of unease, sleep, appetite, ability to concentrate, initiative, emotional involvement, pessimism, and zest for life. The individual is asked to rate each item according to how they have been feeling during the past 3 days, on a scale between 0 and 3. The total score is calculated by summing the answers of the nine items, with higher scores indicating increased severity of symptoms. The MADRS-S does not require a trained person to administer it, and so it would be more appropriate to use in research where there are time constraints or where large samples are being screened. However, unlike the original MADRS, the self-complete version relies on the respondent being literate. Both instruments contain items which could be confounded with the symptoms of diabetes such as difficulties in sleeping and alterations in appetite.

A comparison of the self-report MADRS with the BDI has shown equivalent sensitivity to change during antidepressive treatment in psychiatric patients [103].

Montgomery Asberg Depression Rating Scale – Self-complete version: MADRS-S
Sample questions:
(How you have been feeling during the past 3 days)

Mood

0 I can be either cheerful or sad, depending on the circumstances
0.5
1 I feel a bit low for the most part, though sometimes it eases up a little
1.5
2 I feel thoroughly low and gloomy. Even things that normally cheer me up give me no pleasure
2.5
3 I feel so utterly low and miserable that I can imagine nothing worse

Pessimism

0 I view the future with confidence
0.5
1 Sometimes I am self-critical and think I am less worthy than others

1.5
2 I brood over my failures and feel inferior or worthless, even if others may not agree
2.5
3 Everything seems black to me, and I can see no glimmering of hope. I feel I am thoroughly useless and that there is no chance of forgiveness for the awful things I have done

P Svanborg and M Asberg, 1994

Both the interviewer-based and the self-report scale have been used in research studies, some of which have focused on people with diabetes. Asghar et al. [104] conducted a study of the prevalence of depression in people with diabetes in rural Bangladesh, using the original interviewer-based MADRS. High rates of depressive symptomatology were observed. Similarly high rates of depression were reported in a study comparing people with and without diabetes also using the original MADRS in urban areas of Pakistan [37]. These findings were supported in a previous study in rural Pakistan [105]. In this latter study, the questionnaire was translated into Urdu, although the procedure for doing this is not clear.

The original MADRS has been used in studies of older people and also in people with Parkinson's disease [106]. The Finnish version of MADRS has been used in depressed women with type 2 diabetes [107].

Comparison Between Scales Used to Screen for Depression

When considering which scale to use to screen for depression, there are a number of considerations, one of which is who is going to administer the tool. Some scales, for example, the PHQ-9, can be used without much training as long as the person administering the scale is fully aware that it is only a first-line screen, and further clarification of the symptoms and need for referral and treatment is essential. As we discussed at the beginning of this chapter, many screening instruments have been evaluated according to their sensitivity (how well they perform in terms of identifying all the people with symptoms of depression) and specificity (the ability of a screening tool to identify people with symptoms of depression rather than other psychological morbidities).

For clinical practice, the positive and negative predictive values are also of considerable interest. A low positive predictive value is associated with a high rate of false positives, and a low negative predictive value is associated with a high rate of false negatives. If the positive predictive value is low, the health care professional has to deal with numerous false positives, causing a lot of unnecessary additional diagnostic tests or referrals to mental health specialists.

Table 5.2 Screening performance of screening tools

Screening tool	Sensitivity (%)	Specificity (%)	Positive predictive value (%)	Negative predictive value (%)
BDI	90	84	59	97
BDI-II	87	81	66	83
CES-D	79	89	54	96
PHQ-9	61	94	66	94
WHO-5	100	78	45	100
2 Screening questions	97	67	18	99

Hermanns and Kulzer [24]

A number of research studies have compared different screening tools, in particular, when developing a new tool. For example, the Montgomery Asberg Depression Rating Scale (MADRS) was compared with the Hamilton Rating Scale (HDRS) during its design and initial implementation [100]. Although the two scales were highly correlated, the MADRS was found to be a more precise measure of change than the HDRS. This was in spite of the much smaller number of items on the MADRS (10 compared with 17 on the HDRS). Another study has shown the MADRS to be comparable to the BDI in assessing depression and also to being equivalent in terms of sensitivity to change [103]. The Zung SDS has also been examined in relation to the HDRS [108]. The correlation between these two instruments was found to be high, when comparing their use in patients with diagnosed depressive disorder. The Zung scale was able to distinguish between different levels of symptom severity, and the authors concluded that the ZSDS was a valid and sensitive measure of depressive symptoms.

Another important issue is the screening performance of a scale, that is, how well the scale identifies true cases of depression. Table 5.2 below summarizes the screening performance for case finding of clinical depression of some of the above mentioned screening instruments.

Depression questionnaires like the BDI and CES-D have been shown to have high sensitivity and specificity. Positive predictive values are higher than 50%, and negative predictive values are also good. The questionnaires which are less depression specific like the WHO-5 have a comparable sensitivity to depression questionnaires but a lower specificity. The lower specificity may be due to the fact that these questionnaires measure a broader aspect of psychological well-being or emotional distress. Positive predictive values are lower than 50%. Asking two simple questions about mood or depressed feelings may be, in terms of sensitivity, as effective as using a longer questionnaire. But they have a lower screening performance with regard to specificity or positive predictive values. The relatively smaller screening performance of verbally asked questions may be explained by a varying readiness to speak about emotional problems in patients with diabetes if they are directly asked about depressive feelings.

A further issue is the acceptability of screening for patients and practitioners. This is determined by several aspects regarding performance and content of the questions as well as the time demand for performing a screening measure. Questionnaires asking about diabetes-related distress or general well-being may be better accepted by diabetes patients seeking medical treatment because they may expect to be asked about diabetes-related problems or well-being instead of depressed feelings and suicidal intentions. But this advantage is balanced by a lower specificity, resulting in a higher proportion of false-positive results. For health care professionals, the time needed to score and interpret a screening result is also important.

In our recent research examining the utility of screening tools for measuring depression in people with diabetes, we found wide variations in the prevalence of depression, dependent on the methods used, with good levels of sensitivity and acceptable specificity but low and varying positive predictive values and high negative predictive values for many of the screening tools [8]. However, we raised some concerns with regard to the reported high rate of false positives of many of these screening tools, as indicated by a low positive predictive value. This has important implications for clinical practice as it may lead to inappropriate referrals or follow-up for depression, as well as increasing patient anxiety. We would argue that further work needs to be done in order to tease out whether a particular screening tool is measuring depressive symptoms or symptoms of diabetes so that appropriate care can be offered to individuals with comorbid diabetes and depression.

Conclusions

This chapter has considered the ten most commonly used screening tools for depression in light of the currently available evidence for their utility. Many, if not all, of these instruments have been used in a range of clinical and research settings, albeit with varying success. The evidence suggests that these tools are useful in identifying symptoms of depression, albeit with the caveat that further investigations must be carried out in order to confirm a clinical diagnosis of depression. Screening tools such as those reviewed here are an essential part of that process and, as we have shown, are valid and mostly reliable instruments. Although a small amount of work has been carried out in Europe and Asia, further research does need to be done in order to establish their utility in non-English-speaking populations.

References

1. Lloyd CE. Diabetes and mental health; the problem of co-morbidity. Diabet Med. 2010;27:853–4.
2. Lloyd CE, Pambianco G, Orchard TJ. Does diabetes-related distress explain the presence of depressive symptoms and/or poor self-care in individuals with type 1 diabetes? Diabet Med. 2010;27(2):234–7.

3. Anderson RJ, Freedland KE, Clouse RE, Lustman PJ. The prevalence of co-morbid depression in adults with diabetes. Diabetes Care. 2001;6:1069–78.
4. Ali S, Stone M, Peters J, Davies M, Khunti K. The prevalence of co-morbid depression in adults with type 2 diabetes: a systematic review and meta-analysis. Diabet Med. 2006;23:1165–73.
5. Barnard K, Skinner T, Peveler R. The prevalence of co-morbid depression in adults with type 1 diabetes: systematic literature review. Diabet Med. 2006;23:445–8.
6. Henkel V, Mergl R, Kohnen R, Allgaier AK, Moller HJ, Hegerl U. Use of brief depression screening tools in primary care: consideration of heterogeneity in performance in different patient groups. Gen Hosp Psychiatry. 2004;26:190–8.
7. Babaei F, Mitchell AJ. Screening for depression in medical settings: the case against specific scales. In: Mitchell AJ, Coyne JC, editors. Screening for depression in clinical practice. New York: Oxford University Press; 2010.
8. Roy T, Lloyd CE, Pouwer F, Holt RIG, Sartorius N. Depression screening tools used for measuring depression among people with type 1 and type 2 diabetes; a systematic review. Diabet Med. 2011. doi:10.1111/j.1464–5491.2011.03401.x.
9. Radloff LS. A self-report depression scale for research in the general population. Appl Psychol Meas. 1977;1:385–401.
10. Hermanns N, Kulzer B, Krichbaum M, et al. How to screen for depression and emotional problems in patients with diabetes; comparison of screening characteristics of depression questionnaires, measurement of diabetes specific emotional problems and standard clinical assessment. Diabetologia. 2006;49:469–77.
11. McHale M, Hendrikz J, Dann F, Kenardy J. Screening for depression in patients with diabetes mellitus. Psychosom Med. 2008;70(8):869–74.
12. Fisher L, Skaff MM, Mullan JT, Arean P, Mohr D, Masharani U, Glasgow R, Laurencin G. Clinical depression versus distress among patients with type 2 diabetes. Not just a question of semantics. Diabetes Care. 2007;30:542–8.
13. Pouwer F, Skinner TC, Pibernik-Okanovic M, Beekman ATF, Cradock S, Szabo S, Metelko Z, Snoek FJ. Serious diabetes-specific emotional problems and depression in a Croatian-Dutch-English survey from the Depression in Diabetes Research Consortium. Diabetes Res Clin Pract. 2005;70:166–73.
14. Pibernik-Okanovic M, Begic D, Peros K, Szabo S, Metelko Z. Psychosocial factors contributing to persistent depressive symptoms in type 2 diabetes patients: a Croatian survey from the European Depression in Diabetes Research Consortium. J Diabetes Complications. 2008;22: 246–53.
15. Fisher L, Skaff MM, Mullan JT, Arean P, Glasgow R, Masharani U. A longitudinal study of affective and anxiety disorders, depressive affect and diabetes distress in adults with type 2 diabetes. Diabet Med. 2008;25:1096–101.
16. Golden SH, Lee HB, Schreiner PJ, Roux AD, Fitzpatrick AL, Szklo M, et al. Depression and type 2 diabetes mellitus: the multiethnic study of atherosclerosis. Psychosom Med. 2007;69(6): 529–36.
17. De Groot M, Pinkerman B, Wagner J, Hockman E. Depression treatment and satisfaction in a multicultural sample of type 1 and type 2 diabetic patients. Diabetes Care. 2006;29:549–53.
18. Bisschop MI, Kriegsman DMW, Deeg DJH, Beekman ATF, Van Tilburg W. The longitudinal relation between chronic diseases and depression in older persons in the community: the longitudinal aging study Amsterdam. J Clin Epidermiol. 2004;57:187–94.
19. Geisser ME, Roth RS, Robinson ME. Assessing depression among persons with chronic back pain using the Center for Epidemiological Studies-Depression Scale and the Beck Depression Inventory. Clin J Pain. 1977;13:163–70.
20. Wulsin LR, Singal BM. Do depressive symptoms increase the risk for the onset of coronary disease? A systematic quantitative review. Psychosom Med. 2003;65:201–10.
21. Grzywacz JG, Hovey JD, Seligman LD, Arcury TA, Quandt SA. Evaluating short-form versions of the CES-D for measuring depressive symptoms among immigrants from Mexico. Hispanic J Behav Sci. 2006;28:404–24.

22. Beck AT, Ward CH, Mock J. An inventory for measuring depression. Arch Gen Psychiatry. 1961;4:561–71.
23. Beck AT, Garbin MG. Psychometric properties of the Beck depression inventory: 25 years of evaluation. Clin Psychol Rev. 1988;8:77–100.
24. Beck AT, Steer RA, Brown GK. Beck depression inventory manual. 2nd ed. San Antonio: Psychological Corporation; 1996.
25. Hermanns N, Kulzer B. Diabetes and depression – a burdensome co-morbidity. Eur Endocrinol. 2007;4(2):19–22.
26. Van Tilburg MAL, McCaskill CC, Lane JD, Edwards CL, Bethel A, Feinglos MN, Surwit RS. Depressed mood is a factor in glycemic control in type 1 diabetes. Psychosom Med. 2001;63: 551–5.
27. Palinkas LA, Barrett-Connor E, Wingard DL. Type 2 diabetes and depressive symptoms in older adults: a population based study. Diabet Med. 1991;8:532–9.
28. Gendelman N, Snell-Bergeon JK, McFann K, Kinney G, Wadwa RP, Bishop F, Rewers M, Maahs DM. Prevalence and correlates of depression in individuals with and without type 1 diabetes. Diabetes Care. 2009;32(4):575–9.
29. Lloyd CE, Zgibor J, Wilson RR, Barnett AH, Dyer PH, Orchard TJ. Cross-cultural comparisons of anxiety and depression in adults with type 1 diabetes. Diabetes Metab Res Rev. 2003;19:401–7.
30. Arnau RC, Meagher MW, Norris MP, Bramson R. Psychometric evaluation of the Beck depression inventory-II with primary care medical patients. Health Psychol. 2001;20:112–9.
31. Spitzer RL, Kroenke K, Williams JB, Patient Health Questionnaire Primary Care Study Group. Validation and utility of a self-report version of the PRIME-MD: the PHQ primary care study. JAMA. 1999;282:1737–44.
32. Kroenke K, Spitzer RL, Williams JB. The PHQ-9: validity of a brief depression severity measure. J Gen Intern Med. 2001;16:606–13.
33. Katon W, Von Korff M, Ciechanowski P, Russo J, Lin E, Simon G, Ludman E, Walker E, Bush T, Young B. Behavioural and clinical factors associated with depression among individuals with diabetes. Diabetes Care. 2004;27:914–20.
34. Lowe B, Kroenke K, Herzog W, Grafe K. Measuring depression outcome with a brief self-report instrument: sensitivity to change of the Patient Health Questionnaire. J Affect Disord. 2004;81: 61–6.
35. Katon W, Russo J, Lin EHB, et al. Diabetes and poor disease control: is depression associated with poor adherence or lack of treatment intensification? Psychosom Med. 2009; 71:965–72.
36. Ludman EJ, Katon W, Russo J, von Korff M, Simon G, Ciechanoswski P, et al. Depression and diabetes symptom burden. Gen Hosp Psychiatry. 2004;26:430–6.
37. Faisal F, Asghar S, Zafar M, Hydrie I, Fawwad A, Basit A, Shera S, Hussain A. Depression and diabetes in high-risk urban population of Pakistan. Open Diabet J. 2010;3:1–5. 11876–5246/10 2010 Bentham Open.
38. Lloyd CE, Roy T, Begum S, Mughal S, Barnett AH. Measuring psychological wellbeing in South Asians with diabetes: a qualitative investigation of the PHQ-9 and the WHO-5 as potential screening tools for measuring symptoms of depression. Diabet Med. 2012;29:140–7.
39. Snaith RP, Zigmond AS. Hospital anxiety and depression scale. Acyta Psychiatry Scand. 1983;67:361–70.
40. Lloyd CE, Dyer PH, Barnett AH. Prevalence of symptoms of depression and anxiety in a diabetes clinic population. Diabet Med. 2000;17:198–202.
41. Engum A, Mykletun A, Midthjell K, Holen A, Dahl A. Depression and diabetes: a large population-based study of sociodemographic, lifestyle, and clinical factors associated with depression in type 1 and type 2 diabetes. Diabetes Care. 2005;28:1904–9.
42. Shaban MC, Fosbury J, Kerr D, Cavan DA. The prevalence of depression and anxiety in adults with type 1 diabetes. Diabet Med. 2006;23:1381–4.
43. Montazeri A, Vahdaninia M, Ebrahimi M, Jarvandi S. The Hospital Anxiety and Depression Scale (HADS): translation and validation study of the Iranian version. Health Qual Life Outcomes. 2003;1:14. Online at http://www.hqlo.com/content/1/1/14.

44. Bjelland I, Dahl AA, TangenHaug T, et al. The validity of the Hospital Anxiety and Depression Scale: an updated literature review. J Psychosom Res. 2002;52:69–77.
45. Collins MM, Corcoran P, Perry IJ. Anxiety and depression symptoms in patients with diabetes. Diabet Med. 2009;26:153–61.
46. Dickens CM, Percival C, Mcgowan L, Douglas J, Tomenson B, Cotter L, Heagerty A, Creed FH. The risk factors for depression in first myocardial infarction patients. Psychol Med. 2004;34:1083–92.
47. Carroll BT, Kathol RG, Noyes R, Wald TG, Clamon GH. Screening for depression and anxiety in cancer patients using the Hospital Anxiety and Depression Scale. Gen Hosp Psychiatry. 1993;15:69–74.
48. Tyrer S. Psychiatric assessment of chronic pain. Br J Psychiatry. 1992;160:733–41.
49. Keeley P, Creed F, Tomenson B, Todd C, Borglin G, Dickens C. Psychosocial predictors of health-related quality of life and health service utilisation in people with chronic low back pain. Pain. 2008;135:142–50.
50. Gore M, Brandenburg NA, Dukes E, Hoffman DL, Tai K, Stacey B. Pain severity in diabetic peripheral neuropathy is associated with patient functioning, symptom levels of anxiety and depression, and sleep. J Pain Symp Manage. 2005;30:374–85.
51. Vileikyte L, Leventhal H, Gonzalez JS, Peyrot M, Rubin RR, Ulbrecht JS, et al. Diabetic peripheral neuropathy and depressive symptoms. Diabetes Care. 2005;28:2378–83.
52. Herrmann C. International experiences with the Hospital Anxiety and Depression Scale – a review of validation data and clinical results. J Psychosom Res. 1997;42:17–41.
53. Michopoulos I, Douzenis A, Kalkavoura C, Christodoulou C, Michalopoulou P, Kalemi G, Fineti K, Patapis P, Protopapas K, Lykouras L. Hospital anxiety and depression scale (HADS): validation in a Greek general hospital sample. Ann Gen Psychiatry. 2008;7:4. doi:10.1186/1744–859X-7–4.
54. Zung WWK. A self-rating depression scale. Arch Gen Psychiatry. 1965;12:63–70.
55. Campo-Arias A, Dlaz-Martinez LA, Rueda-Jaimes GE, Cadena LDP, Hernandez NL. Validation of the Zung self-rating depression scale among the Columbian general population. Soc Behav Personal. 2006;34:87–94.
56. Yoshida S, Hirai M, Suzuki S, Awata S, Oka Y. Neuropathy is associated with depression independently of health-related quality of life in Japanese patients with diabetes. Psychiatry Clin Neurosci. 2009;63(1):65–72.
57. Xu L, Ren J, Cheng M, Tang K, Dong M, Hou X, Sun L, Chen L. Depressive symptoms and risk factors in Chinese persons with type 2 diabetes. Arch Med Res. 2004;35(4):301–7.
58. Yu R, Y-Hua L, Hong L. Depression in newly diagnosed type 2 diabetes. Int J Diabet Dev Countries. 2010;30(2):102–4.
59. Yang J, Li S, Zheng Y. Predictors of depression in Chinese community-dwelling people with type 2 diabetes. J Clin Nurs. 2009;18(9):1295–304.
60. Rajala U, Keinanen-Kiukaanniemi S. Non-insulin-dependent diabetes mellitus and depression in a middle-aged Finnish population. Soc Psychiatry Psychiatr Epidemiol. 1997;32:363–7.
61. Kawakami N, Takatsuka N, Shimizu H, Ishibashi H. Depressive symptoms and occurrence of type 2 diabetes among Japanese men. Diabetes Care. 1999;22:1071–6.
62. Zung WWK. The depression status inventory: an adjunct to the self-rating depression scale. J Clin Psychol. 1972;28:539–43.
63. Romano C, De Giovanni L, Santoro PE, Spataro M. The relationship between mobbing and depression syndrome in the female working population of service industry: the problem statement and the prevention strategies in Sicilian environment. G Ital Med Lav Ergon. 2007;29(3):675–8.
64. Kiljunen M, Sulkava R, Niinistö L, Polvikoski T, Verkkoniemi A, Halonen P. Depression measured by the Zung depression status inventory is very rare in a Finnish population aged 85 years and over. Int Psychogeriatr. 1997;9(3):359–68.
65. Lupsakko T, Mäntyjärvi M, Kautiainen H, Sulkava R. Combined hearing and visual impairment and depression in a population aged 75 years and older. Int J Geriatr Psychiatry. 2002;17(9):808–13.
66. Funke HJ, Holtmann W, Ismail S, Jansen W, Leonhardt KF, Muth H, Omer LM, O'Connolly M, Ramm H. Double-blind comparison of diclofensine with nomifensine in outpatients with dysphoric mood. Pharmacopsychiatry. 1986;19(3):120–3.

67. Ware JE. SF-36 health survey. Manual and interpretation guide. Boston: The Health Institute; 1993.
68. Hemingway H, Nicholson A, Stafford M, Roberts R, Marmot M. The impact of socioeconomic status on health functioning as assessed by the SF-36 questionnaire: the Whitehall study. Am J Public Health. 1997;87:1484–90.
69. Goldney RD, Phillips PJ, Fisher LJ, Wilson DH. Diabetes, depression and quality of life. Diabetes Care. 2004;27:1066–70.
70. Lange LJ, Piette JD. Perceived health status and perceived diabetes control: psychological indicators and accuracy. J Psychosom Res. 2005;58:129–37.
71. Claiborne N, Massaro E. Mental quality of life: an indicator of unmet needs in patients with diabetes. Soc Work Health Care. 2000;32:25–43.
72. Ware JE, Kosinski M, Keller SD. A 12-item short-form health survey: construction of scales and preliminary tests of reliability. Med Care. 1996;34:220–33.
73. Ware JE, Kosinski M, Turner-Bowker DM, Gandek B. User's manual for the SF-12v2™ health survey. Boston: QualityMetric Incorporated Lincoln, and Health Assessment Lab; 2007.
74. Bair MJ, Brizendine EJ, Ackermann RT, Shen C, Kroenke K, Marrero DG. Prevalence of pain and association with quality of life, depression and glycaemic control in patients with diabetes. Diabet Med. 2010;27:57–584.
75. Hamilton M. A rating scale for depression. J Neurol Neurosurg Psychiatry. 1960;23:56–62.
76. Williams JB. A structured interview guide for the Hamilton Depression Rating Scale. Arch Gen Psychiatry. 1988;45:742–7.
77. Kokoszka A, Pouwer F, Jodko A, Radzio R, Mucko P, Bienkowska J, et al. Serious diabetes-specific emotional problems in patients with type 2 diabetes who have different levels of comorbid depression: a Polish study from the European Depression in Diabetes (EDID) Research Consortium. Eur Psychiatry. 2009;24(7):425–30.
78. Agbir TM, Audu MD, Adebowale TO, Goar SG. Depression among medical outpatients with diabetes: a cross-sectional study at Jos University Teaching Hospital, Jos, Nigeria. Ann Afr Med. 2010;9(1):5–10.
79. Olden M, Rosenfeld B, Pessin H, Breitbart W. Measuring depression at the end of life: is the Hamilton Depression Rating Scale a valid instrument? Assessment. 2009;16:43–54.
80. Bagby RM, Ryder AG, Schuller DR, Marchall MB. The Hamilton Depression Rating Scale: has the gold standard become a lead weight? Am J Psychiatry. 2004;161:2163–77.
81. Goldberg DP, Gater R, Sartorius N, Ustun TB, Piccinelli M, Gureje O, Rutter C. The validity of two versions of the GHQ in the WHO study of mental illness in general health care. Psychol Med. 1997;27:191–7.
82. Jacob KS, Bhugra D, Mann AH. The validation of the 12-item General Health Questionnaire among ethnic Indian women living in the United Kingdom. Psychol Med. 1997;27:1215–7.
83. Bhui K, Bhugra D, Goldberg D. Cross-cultural validity of the Amritsar Depression Inventory and the General Health Questionnaire amongst English and Punjabi primary care attenders. Soc Psychiatry Psychiatr Epidemiol. 2000;35:248–54.
84. Esteban y Peña MM, Hernandez Barrera V, Fernández Cordero X, de Gil Miguel A, Rodríguez Pérez M, Lopez-de Andres A, et al. Self-perception of health status, mental health and quality of life among adults with diabetes residing in a metropolitan area. Diabetes Metab. 2010;36(4):305–11.
85. Pirkola S, Saarni S, Suvisaari J, Elovainio M, Partonen T, Aalto AM, et al. General health and quality-of-life measures in active, recent, and comorbid mental disorders: a population-based health 2000 study. Compr Psychiatry. 2009;50(2):108–14.
86. Bech P. Rating scales for psychopathology, health status and quality of life. A compendium on documentation in accordance with the DSM-III-R and WHO systems. Berlin: Springer; 1993.
87. Bech P, Olsen RL, Kjoller M, Rasmussen NK. Measuring well-being rather than the absence of distress symptoms: a comparison of the SF-36 Mental Health subscale and the WHO-Five Well-Being Scale. Int J Methods Psychiatr Res. 2003;12:85–91.

88. Bech P. Measuring the dimensions of psychological general well-being by the WHO-5. QoL Newsl. 2004;32:15–6.
89. Aujla N, Abrams KR, Davies MJ, Taub N, Skinner TC, Khunti K. The prevalence of depression in white-European and South-Asian people with impaired glucose regulation and screen-detected type 2 diabetes mellitus. PLoS One. 2009;4(11):e7755.
90. Awata S, Bech P, Yoshida S, Hirai M, Suzuki S, Yamashita M, Ohara A, Hinokio Y, Matsuoka H, Oka Y. Reliability and validity of the Japanese version of the World Health Organization-Five Well-Being Index in the context of detecting depression in diabetic patients. Psychiatry Clin Neurosci. 2007;61:112–9.
91. Papanas N, Tsapas A, Papatheodorou K, Papazoglou D, Bekiari E, Sariganni M, Paletas K, Maltezos E. Glycaemic control is correlated with Well-Being Index (WHO-5) in subjects with type 2 diabetes. Exp Clin Endocrinol Diabetes. 2010;118:364–7.
92. Saipanish R, Lotrakul M, Sumrithe S. Reliability and validity of the Thai version of the WHO-Five Well-Being Index in primary care patients. Psychiatry Clin Neurosci. 2009;63:141–6.
93. Sibai AM, Chaaya M, Tohme RA, Mahfoud Z, Al-Amin H. Validation of the Arabic version of the 5-item WHO Well Being Index in elderly population. Int J Geriatr Psychiatry. 2009;24:106–7.
94. Birket-Smith M, Rasmussen A. Screening for mental disorders in cardiology outpatients. Nord J Psychiatry. 2008;62:147–50.
95. Bech P, Rasmussen NA, Olsen LR, Noerholm V, Abildgaard W. The sensitivity and specificity of the Major Depression Inventory, using the Present State Examination as the index of diagnosis validity. J Affect Disord. 2001;66:159–64.
96. Fountoulakis KN, Iacovides A, Kleanthous S, Samolis S, Gougoulia K, Kaprinis SG, Bech P. Reliability, validity and psychometric properties of the Greek translation of the Major Depression Inventory. BMC Psychiatry. 2003;3:2.
97. Olsen LR, Jensen DV, Noerholm V, Martiny K, Bech P. The internal and external validity of the Major Depression Inventory in measuring depressive states. Psychol Med. 2003;33:351–6.
98. Bech P. Health-related quality of life measurements in the assessment of pain clinic results. Acta Anaesthesiol Scand. 1999;43:893–6.
99. Bech P, Wermuth L. Applicability and validity of the Major Depression Inventory in patients with Parkinsons disease. Nord Psykiatr Tidsskr. 1998;52:305–9.
100. Montgomery SA, Asberg M. A new depression scale designed to be sensitive to change. Br J Psychiatry. 1979;134:382–9.
101. Zimmerman M, Chelminski I, Posternak M. A review of studies of the Hamilton depression rating scale in health controls: implications for the definition of remission in treatment studies of depression. J Nerv Ment Dis. 2004;192:595–601.
102. Fantino B, Moore N. The self-reported Montgomery-Asberg depression rating scale is a useful evaluative tool in major depressive disorder. BMC Psychiatry. 2009;9:26.
103. Svanborg P, Asberg M. A new self-rating scale for depression and anxiety states based on the comprehensive psychopathological rating scale. Acta Psychiatr Scand. 1994;89:21–8.
104. Asghar S, Hussain A, Ali S, Khan A, Magnusson A. Prevalence of depression and diabetes: a population-based study from rural Bangladesh. Diabet Med. 2007;24:872–7.
105. Zahid N, Asghar S, Claussen B, Hussain A. Depression and diabetes in a rural community in Pakistan. Diabetes Res Clin Pract. 2008;79:124–7.
106. Tandberg E, Larsen JP, Aarsland D, Cummings JL. The occurrence of depression in Parkinson's disease. A community-based study. Arch Neurol. 1996;53:175–9.
107. Paile-Hyvärinen M, Wahlbeck K, Eriksson JG. Quality of life and metabolic status in mildly depressed women with type 2 diabetes treated with paroxetine: a single-blind randomised placebo controlled trial. BMC Fam Pract. 2003;4:7. Epub 2003 May 14.
108. Biggs JT, Wylie LT, Ziegler VE. Validity of the Zung self-rating depression scale. Br J Psychiatry. 1978;132:381–5.

Part II
Screening for Depression in Different Settings

Chapter 6
Measuring Depression in Children and Young People

Korey K. Hood, Diana M. Naranjo, and Katharine Barnard

Abstract Diabetes is not simply a public health burden but rather a very personal daily challenge for people living with the disease. Diabetes and its management impose additional cognitive and emotional burdens that can take the form of increased vigilance to dietary intake, symptom monitoring, and frustrations with blood glucose excursions. For the child or young person with diabetes, this daily challenge is superimposed on physical development, competing priorities with age-appropriate activities, and a family environment that is constantly adapting to diabetes and its management. For these reasons, the child with diabetes can experience difficulties in psychological adjustment, and identification, prevention, and treatment of these difficulties are essential. Likewise, those administering to the child or young person, namely, parents or other family members, may also experience problems from a psychological functioning standpoint. This chapter aims to provide a context to understanding the potential difficulties, how to measure areas of risk including depression and anxiety, and how to use that information in clinical practice. Recommendations are provided in order to screen for psychological adjustment difficulties, particularly depression, and how to respond to positive screenings and potential referral options for intervention.

K.K. Hood, Ph.D. (✉)
Department of Pediatrics, University of California San Francisco,
San Francisco, CA, USA
e-mail: hoodk@peds.ucsf.edu

D.M. Naranjo, Ph.D.
Division of General Pediatrics, Department of Pediatrics,
University of California San Francisco, San Francisco, CA, USA
e-mail: naranjod@peds.ucsf.edu

K. Barnard, Ph.D.
Faculty of Medicine, University of Southampton, Hampshire, UK
e-mail: k.barnard@soton.ac.uk

C.E. Lloyd et al. (eds.), *Screening for Depression and Other Psychological Problems in Diabetes*,
DOI 10.1007/978-0-85729-751-8_6,

Keywords Children • Young people • Type 1 diabetes • Psychological screening Psychological adjustment • Diabetes management • Pediatric diabetes • Interventions • Depression • Diabetes burnout

Mental Health Disorders in Children and Young People

Community and regional surveys within the United States (US) indicate that about one in every 3–4 children experiences a mental disorder [1–7] and that about one in ten children has a serious emotional disturbance [8, 9]. Although slightly lower, statistics based on US national samples are still disturbingly high. A recent article based upon the US National Health and Nutrition Examination Survey shows that in young people aged 8–15 years old, attention-deficit/hyperactivity disorder is the most common disorder at 8.6%, followed by mood disorders at 3.7%, conduct disorder at 2.1%, panic disorder or generalized anxiety disorder at 0.7%, and eating disorders at 0.1% [10]. Certain disorders appeared to be qualified by gender with boys having roughly two times greater prevalence of attention-deficit/hyperactivity disorder than girls, and the reverse in mood disorder. Other disorders like anxiety disorders and conduct disorder do not vary across gender among youth. In another US national survey of older adolescents aged 13–18 [11], the most common conditions are anxiety disorders (31.9%), followed by behavior disorders (19.1%), mood disorders (14.3%), and substance use disorders (11.4%), with approximately 40% of participants meeting criteria more than one mental health disorder. Similar rates have been observed in the UK, with one in ten children between the ages of 5 and 15 having a clinically diagnosable mental disorder (including anxiety and depression) that is associated with "considerable distress and substantial interference with personal functions" such as family and social relationships, their capacity to cope with day-to-day stresses and life challenges, and their learning [12]. Prevalence rates vary according to gender, with problems more common in boys than girls, and age, with problems more common among 11–15-year-olds than 5–10-year-olds [13].

Prevalence rates of depression and other emotional problems among children and adolescents with diabetes are alarmingly higher than in the general population samples. Clinically elevated depressive symptoms are present in 15–25% of adolescents with type 1 diabetes [14–16], and these symptoms are associated with poor self-care, suboptimal glycemic control, and recurrent diabetic ketoacidosis [17–20]. In addition to increased risk for anxiety and depressive symptoms, adolescents with type 1 diabetes are at increased risk for poor coping and problem-solving skills [21, 22], poor self-care [23, 24], and negative diabetes-specific health outcomes such as suboptimal glycemic control and recurrent diabetic ketoacidosis [25–27].

Why Difficulties in Psychological Adjustment Occur

Most cases of diabetes in children and young people are type 1 diabetes. For the better part of two decades, there has been a steady increase in the incidence of type 1 diabetes in children, giving clinicians, researchers, and policy makers reason to call this an epidemic [28]. Type 1 diabetes is typically diagnosed in late childhood or early adolescence; however, there is increasing incidence in young children. This autoimmune disease is characterized by the insufficient or complete lack of insulin production in the body. Consequently, the management of type 1 diabetes includes the coordination of insulin dosing and administration with other critical variables: blood glucose levels, dietary intake, and physical activity. The effective management of this complex and demanding management regimen requires behavioral and emotional health, for both the child and family members involved in daily diabetes care [29]. The mental and physical health risks of type 1 diabetes add to its already staggering economic burden; the annual cost of diabetes in the US for direct medical care exceeds $116 billion, and individuals with diabetes have twice the health-care costs of their peers without diabetes [30, 31].

Of note, fewer children and young people have type 2 diabetes [32, 33]. Type 2 diabetes is characterized by insulin resistance, and treatment can involve oral medications (e.g., metformin) and/or insulin but almost always includes lifestyle changes in the form of reduced sedentary behavior, increased physical activity, and healthy eating. Given that the largest proportion of diabetes in children and young people is type 1 diabetes, much of the focus of this chapter will be on psychological functioning and measurement in those youth and families. As appropriate, evidence on pediatric type 2 diabetes will be noted in the chapter.

Just like the multifactorial etiology of pediatric diabetes, there are multiple contributors to the psychological functioning of the child or young person with diabetes. Appropriate adjustment to diabetes and being able to put the disease into context with other life priorities are essential to avoid being overwhelmed by the condition and feeling controlled by it. Increased treatment flexibility and greater access to education about self-management have enabled people to fit diabetes into their lives rather than vice versa and maintain a balance between respecting the severity of the condition and enjoying both independence and a good quality of life. However, this seems to be more difficult for children and young people than for adults with diabetes [23, 34].

Part of this can be attributed to the cognitive development of the child or young person; they may not be able to understand how carrying out a behavior to manage diabetes makes another desirable activity easier. For example, playing sports and operating at an optimal level will be hindered by wide-ranging blood glucose levels, but most young people do not want to stop these activities to check blood glucose levels and correct a high or low level. Diabetes and its management are often seen as a nuisance in these situations and may lead to feelings of frustration and anger with diabetes. From that social perspective, having diabetes has the potential to set the child or young person aside from "normal" society and imperceptibly outside the social constructs of what it is to be healthy. Societal norms bring with them prejudices and arbitrary or erroneous rules about how to behave. People with diabetes often report the stigma associated with the condition, affecting not only health but also social functioning [35]. Other contributors to the development of difficulties in psychological adjustment are likely to include the relentless nature of diabetes management and having to do tasks multiple times daily, feeling that other age-appropriate priorities cannot be met in the presence of diabetes, and the cognitive demands of near-constant vigilance to food, blood glucose levels, and activity levels.

A Note About the Family

Diabetes is a demanding, long-term condition that impacts not only the life of the individual but also on the lives of other family members. Type 1 diabetes, for example, has often been characterized as a "family disease" given both its impact on the family and the family's role in diabetes management [36, 37]. For young children (~8 and under), most care comes from parents who administer or oversee treatment [38]. Children ages 9–12 often begin to take on more responsibility for diabetes management, although parents or other adults are still supervising treatment. In the teenage years (13 and above), there is ideally a negotiation that occurs between parents and adolescents about the responsibility for diabetes; however, communication problems and increased family conflict often occur [39, 40] jeopardizing the successful execution of management tasks.

The role of parenting in caring for children with type 1 diabetes is vital, with parents being crucial to promoting positive disease adaptation and health outcomes [41, 42]. Successful diabetes management, however, may come with negative consequences to parents' own well-being. Diabetes-related management practices, time demands, finances, social support, independence, stigma, and concern for the future must all be balanced with achieving optimal glycemic control and quality of life for the child or young person. Further, the quality of life of family members is affected by a child's diabetes, with family members reporting limitations and anxiety associated with living with someone with diabetes [43].

The organization and execution of diabetes management for a child or young person are carried out in the context of the family, and the psychological functioning of those family members affects and is affected by diabetes and its management. In other words, the child, diabetes, and the family are interconnected. In addition to the family, a full conceptualization of the context of a child or young person's psychological adjustment and diabetes management has to include consideration of culture and gender.

Screening for Aspects of Psychological Functioning: Depression

Nature of Depression

For the purpose of specificity within this chapter, we rely on the World Health Organization (WHO) and its definition, which is: "a common mental disorder that presents with depressed mood, loss of interest or pleasure, feelings of guilt or low self-worth, disturbed sleep or appetite, low energy, and poor concentration" [44]. Depression is a nondiscriminatory disease in that it affects people of all genders, ages, and backgrounds. Ranging from subclinical depressive symptomatology, at its worst depression can lead to suicide, contributing to an estimated 850,000 deaths worldwide every year [44].

The definition of depression does not change for people with diabetes, but there are a number of factors to consider. First, as noted earlier, there are elevated rates of depression in adults, young people, and children with diabetes compared to individuals without diabetes [14, 45, 46]. The reasons for this are complex, but most attribute the higher rates in people with diabetes to the burden of living with a chronic disease and its unrelenting management. Much of the work in this area has focused on type 1 diabetes, and there are consistent findings in this type of diabetes. There are emerging data in children and young people with type 2 diabetes, some of which does not support the data from adults with type 2 diabetes. Recently, results were published from baseline data of a large clinical trial in the US, the TODAY study, which indicated that rates in youth with type 2 diabetes are slightly lower than youth with type 1 diabetes and higher for girls than boys [47]. This overlaps with findings reported from the SEARCH for Diabetes in Youth study, which showed relatively few elevations in depressive symptoms in this large sample, except for males with type 2 diabetes and female participants with multiple medical comorbidities [48].

Screening for Depression

The major diabetes organizations around the world, including the International Society for Pediatric and Adolescent Diabetes (ISPAD) and the American Diabetes Association (ADA), have advocated for screening for depression in pediatric patients [29, 49]. However, little systematic screening takes place in pediatric diabetes centers worldwide. This is due to a number of factors dealing with inadequacy of time to screen and staff to respond to positive screenings, disruptions in clinic flow, and uncertainty about the best methods for screening. Below, we make suggestions as to how to screen for depression in children and young people which we view as an essential aspect of diabetes care. There are two legitimate options: asking a series of questions or administering a brief questionnaire. As discussed elsewhere in this book, there are two screening questions used in the UK which we feel are a valuable starting point [50, 51]:

Screening questions used to open a clinical discussion about depression
"During the past month have you often been bothered by feeling down, depressed, or hopeless?"
"During the past month have you often been bothered by little interest or pleasure in doing things?"

Although these two questions have been well validated in adults, their validity in children and young people has not yet been strongly established. Furthermore, one important component of depression in young people that might be missed by only using these two questions is that of symptoms of irritability. Notwithstanding these limitations, if those two questions are answered affirmatively, a series of follow-up questions can be asked about what those feelings were like, any problems in functioning because of them (e.g., could not focus at school or did not check blood glucose levels as much), and if they sought help. However, the best option is to make a referral to a mental health professional. This may be a social worker, counselor, psychologist, or psychiatrist working in a diabetes center or with diabetes patients.

A more systematic approach is administering a validated self-report questionnaire. There are two that are used often in mental health assessment and treatment and have been administered widely in pediatric diabetes studies. They are the Children's Depression Inventory (CDI) and the Center for Epidemiologic Studies – Depression (CES-D) scale. The Beck Depression Inventory – II (BDI-II) can also be used for young people 13 and above.

The CDI is a self-report questionnaire consisting of 27 items rated from 0 (no symptom) to 2 (distinct symptom) [52]. Items on the CDI cut across multiple types of symptoms (e.g., sadness, low self-esteem) and functional areas (e.g., not having friends, schoolwork is not as good as it was before, and arguing with others). The child or young person is asked to endorse one of three responses for each of the 27 items. An example is choosing among "I am sad once in a while," "I am sad many times," and "I am sad all the time." Other items address feeling tired and feelings of isolation.

CDI scores can range from 0 to 54 with a clinical cutoff score of 13 or higher indicative of elevated depressive symptoms and suggestive of further evaluation [52]. The CDI is copyrighted, has a cost, and is published by Multi-Health Systems Inc. in the US. Caregivers can also provide a proxy report of the child's depressive symptoms on the 17-item parent version (CDI:P). A score of 17 and higher is indicative of significant child depressive symptomatology.

On the CDI, item #9 assesses suicidal ideation and should always be inspected for any response other than "I do not think about killing myself." A plan for responding to positive endorsements on this item should be in place when using the CDI.

The 20-item CES-D [53] is widely used, and large sample normative data and clinical cutoff scores (≥16) are available [53]. Respondents endorse items on a scale from 0 (not experiencing that symptom) to 3 (experiencing that symptom all the time) over the past week. This has been used in pediatric patients, although its original use was with adults. It is the measure used in the large prospective study, SEARCH for Diabetes in Youth [48]. While SEARCH has the primary aims of documenting the prevalence, incidence, and course of diabetes in 5 racial/ethnic groups in the US [32, 54], many other aspects of living with diabetes, such as depression and quality of life, are also assessed in these children and young people with diabetes. While strict cutoffs for pediatric patients have not been identified in any study including SEARCH, a score of 16 and above can be used to refer for further evaluation. The CES-D is free and accessible on the internet (search by name of measure, not just CES-D). It has been translated in to multiple languages.

Sample CES-D items
"During the past week I was bothered by things that usually don't bother me"
"During the past week I felt depressed"
"During the past week I had restless sleep"
"During the past week I talked less than usual"

After the method for screening has been identified, it is important to have a protocol for handling positive screenings. For example, scores above a certain threshold will always be referred to a mental health provider, while "subclinical" scores may just be watched and reviewed at the next visit. As noted above, a protocol for responding to positive suicidal ideation is also necessary. This may involve an immediate evaluation by a mental health provider or referral to an emergency department or crisis unit. In these cases, we recommend erring on the side of caution even if you suspect a false positive.

Feedback to the patient and family and a well-documented plan are also necessary. Patients and their families should be told what their scores or responses mean and where they fall compared to other youth. For example, "you obtained a score of 15 on the CDI and a score of 13 or above tells us that it would be helpful to talk with a mental health professional to find out more and possibly figure out a way to help you." Having patients and families leave the clinic visit with a written-out plan will assist with overburdening patients to memorize the plan. Of note, however, is a recent report that documents that this is not sufficient to improve depression, at least in adults [55]. Thus, it is important to just see this as a first step to set up the patient and family for more intensive assessment and treatment.

Screening for Subclinical Depression and Diabetes Burnout

Nature of Subclinical Depression and Burnout

Subclinical depression is a term used when an individual presents with depressive symptoms but does not meet the criteria for a diagnosis of clinical depression. Recent reports note that approximately one-third of people with type 1 diabetes and 37–43% of people with type 2 diabetes report symptoms of depression [56, 57]. These rates were far higher than the proportion of people who had been given an actual diagnosis of clinical depression [45]. Rather than receiving treatment for depression, however, such individuals often have to cope with their symptoms alone. The impact on family, social life, and overall quality of life remains unknown to a large extent and is an area where further research is clearly needed. When screening for depression or psychological distress in pediatric patients with diabetes, we recommend that scores just below a "clinical" threshold be monitored closely at follow-up visits. The natural course of depression is to worsen [58]; thus, close follow-up and possible prevention efforts are warranted.

Alternatively, research has indicated that another group exists. This consists of a substantial proportion of individuals who are not depressed and do not report depressive symptomatology yet still feel unable to cope with their diabetes. It has been suggested that these people are experiencing diabetes-related distress or are "burned out" by their diabetes. Diabetes burnout occurs when a person feels "overwhelmed by diabetes and by the frustrating burden of diabetes self-care"[59]. These emotions may be different to feelings of depression, but because of their diabetes-specific nature, they are often just as destructive and have implications for diabetes care.

Screening for Diabetes Burnout

It is important to assess for the following symptoms of diabetes burnout during routine visits:

- Feeling overwhelmed and defeated by diabetes
- Feeling angry about diabetes, frustrated by the self-care regimen, and/or having other strong negative feelings about diabetes
- Feeling that diabetes is controlling their life
- Worrying about not taking care of diabetes well enough yet unable, unmotivated, or unwilling to change
- Avoiding any/all diabetes-related tasks that might give feedback about consequences of poor control
- Feeling alone and isolated with diabetes

There are several measures that can be used to examine diabetes burnout, although most are adapted from use in adult populations. They include the Diabetes Distress Scale (DDS) and the Problem Areas in Diabetes (PAID) scale, both developed out of the work of Polonsky et al. [60, 61]. There is a downward extension of the PAID for teens that was recently validated [62]. This measure contains 26 items and is completed on a 6-point Likert scale. It has strong reliability and validity and provides a snapshot of the areas about diabetes that are most distressing to teens.

Sample items from the PAID for teenagers
Feeling "burned out" by the constant effort to manage diabetes
Feeling that I am not checking my blood sugars often enough
Feeling that my friends or family act like "diabetes police" (e.g., nag about eating properly, checking blood sugars, not trying hard enough)
Feeling I must be perfect in my diabetes management
Fitting my diabetes regimen into my day when I'm away from home (e.g., school, work, etc.)

Likewise, the Blood Glucose Monitoring and Communication (BGMC) survey can be used to specifically assess frustration and anger with blood glucose monitoring [63]. This is just an 8-item measure and can be completed by the child as well as the parent. It is depicted below:

The Blood Glucose Monitoring and Communication Survey [63]
1. When my blood sugar is high, I get upset thinking that I will be blamed for something I ate.
2. When my blood sugar is high, I feel scared.
3. When my blood sugar is high, I feel frustrated.
4. I am upset when I have high blood sugar.
5. I feel angry when my blood sugar is high.
6. I feel frustrated when I have low blood sugar.
7. When my blood sugar is high, I feel guilty.
8. When my blood sugar is low, I feel scared.

Finally, there is another adaptation of the PAID's theme of burnout for parents which includes 20 items and provides an indication of areas parents of children and young people with diabetes find most distressing [64]. Items are similar to the PAID items for teens, but focus on the parental perception of the role diabetes plays in daily activities and quality of life. Most of these measures are accessible and free by contacting the corresponding authors of the cited articles.

Screening for Aspects of Psychological Functioning: Anxiety

Nature of Anxiety

In contrast to depression, much less work has been done on the nature of anxiety in children and young people with diabetes as well as the relationship between anxiety and diabetes management and health outcomes. However, several studies show that worries about diabetes and negative affect (e.g., state and trait anxiety) negatively impact on disease management and glycemic control in children and young people [65–67]. In adults with type 1 diabetes, anxiety has been linked with less frequent blood glucose monitoring and suboptimal glycemic control [68].

Interestingly, depression and anxiety are often comorbid conditions in children and young people [69], which can complicate the clinical picture and context. There is also the potential that the symptoms of these two conditions may act in opposite directions with regard to diabetes management and control. Thus, we recommend assessing anxiety and doing so separately from depression.

Screening for Anxiety

The nature of anxiety and its symptomatology suggest that surveying pediatric patients for the following may be clinically informative:

- Constant worries or fears that intrude on the patient's ability to focus or concentrate
- Frequent worries or fears about developing diabetes complications, separate from diabetes burnout or distress
- Hypervigilance on "perfect" diabetes control or an overly perfectionist attitude in general

Screening for anxiety in children and young people with diabetes can also include the use of well-validated surveys. One in particular is the State-Trait Anxiety Inventory (STAI) for children [66, 70]. The STAI has 40 items with 20 each devoted to either state or trait anxiety. The state items use "I feel" as the stem, and then each of the 20 items has three options.

Sample items from the STAI state scale
I feel VERY CALM, CALM, or NOT CALM
I feel VERY WORRIED, WORRIED, or NOT WORRIED
I feel VERY NICE, NICE, or NOT NICE
I feel VERY RELAXED, RELAXED, or NOT RELAXED
I feel VERY CHEERFUL, CHEERFUL, or NOT CHEERFUL

The STAI trait items are responded to as "hardly ever," "sometimes," or "often." For example, "I feel like crying" or "I am shy" would have to be endorsed as hardly ever, sometimes, or often. The STAI does not specifically address anxiety symptoms within the context of diabetes; however, understanding whether anxiety symptoms are rooted in general areas or are diabetes-specific may be particularly helpful in treatment planning and delivery. It may be equally useful to determine types of anxiety (e.g., fears, phobias, obsessions/compulsions) and symptoms (e.g., difficulty concentrating, fatigue, forgetfulness) that interfere with diabetes management and glycemic control. A large component of the anxiety experienced by children and young people with diabetes and their parents has to do with hypoglycemia. This is addressed in the next section.

Screening for Fear of Hypoglycemia (Children and Parents)

Nature of the Fear of Hypoglycemia

Since the Diabetes Control and Complications Trial (DCCT) showed that tighter control reduces complication rates [71], there has been more emphasis on intensified insulin therapy. One of the risks of intensified insulin therapy and tighter control is an increased risk of hypoglycemia. Children and young people learn quickly that hypoglycemic episodes are physically aversive, potentially dangerous, and a source of possible social embarrassment [72]. Parents also acknowledge significant anxiety about the occurrence of hypoglycemic episodes and may maintain marginally elevated blood glucose levels and engage in premature treatment of apparent hypoglycemia [73, 74]. At times, the associated risks of long-term complications can be overshadowed by short-term goals to avoid hypoglycemia.

The clinical picture is quite concerning as parents have a number of diabetes-specific worries and anxieties that include fear of hypoglycemia and associated seizures both during the day and at night, anxiety associated with frequent blood glucose monitoring, fear of "not being there" despite daily management being relentless, and fear that others, such as babysitters and teachers, will be unable to provide appropriate care for their child. Experiencing hypoglycemia at some point in time after diagnosis and engaging in subsequent avoidance behaviors contribute to the problem. Paradoxically, chronically higher HbA1c levels are associated with the signs of acute hypoglycemia presenting at higher blood glucose levels. This means hypoglycemic signs can be present when the patient is actually hyperglycemic and not hypoglycemic. Thus, parents engage in further avoidance behaviors, leading to even higher HbA1c levels, causing a spiraling effect of worsening diabetes control. These behaviors can be either conscious or subconscious with fear a strong motivating factor to maintain such maladaptive coping despite the long-term risks.

A recent literature review of the contributing factors to parental fear reported that mothers of young children with type 1 diabetes reported greater fear of hypoglycemia and took more steps to avoid it than fathers did [74]. However, mothers and fathers reported the same level of worry about hypoglycemia. Fathers, however, experience greater levels of parenting stress and have lower confidence in their ability to manage their child's diabetes, reporting greater anxiety and increased hopelessness than mothers. In a study cited in this review, half of parents reported the child experiencing an episode of hypoglycemia 3–5 times per week [75]. However, the *severity* of hypoglycemia seems more important in causing fear than *frequency*, especially in parents whose child had experienced a hypoglycemic seizure. Mothers whose children had a history of passing out experienced far greater worry than mothers whose children had never lost consciousness. Furthermore, children who had experienced a seizure with loss of consciousness had a significantly higher percentage of blood glucose levels above the desired target range than young children with no history of seizures, which suggests that parents of these children are indeed allowing higher than desired blood glucose levels to avoid hypoglycemia.

Screening for Fear of Hypoglycemia

The first step in screening is ensuring that questions are asked about the frequency and severity of hypoglycemia, as is typical of clinical visit dialogue, but also asking a specific question about fears. It may help to ask for specific examples of hypoglycemic episodes and probe about thoughts and feelings during and after the event. It is also helpful to ask about any change in behaviors associated with that event or an ongoing fear.

More information can be obtained about fears in this area by having patients and parents complete surveys. This will provide richer data for the clinician to consider in treatment planning. The most widely used measures are the fear of hypoglycemia scales [76–78]. There are forms for children and young people, parents, and adults with type 1 diabetes. All are well validated and contain items that are specific to situations (e.g., sleeping, driving) as well as more general experiences with hypoglycemia.

Sample items from the fear of hypoglycemia scale for children					
Worry: Below is a list of worries children with diabetes sometimes have about low blood sugar. Circle the number that best describes YOU.					
0 = NEVER 1 = RARELY 2 = SOMETIMES 3 = OFTEN 4 = ALMOST ALWAYS					
11. Not recognizing that my blood sugar is low	0	1	2	3	4
14. Having a hypo while asleep	0	1	2	3	4
15. Embarrassing myself because of low blood sugar	0	1	2	3	4
16. Having a hypo while I am by myself	0	1	2	3	4

Further, it may be important to assess parental anxiety and depression, possibly with the CES-D or STAI scales, and pair those results with the fear surveys. It is critical to understand the pervasiveness of these fears, worries, and distress as it relates to diabetes management and control.

Screening for Aspects of Psychological Functioning: Alcohol Use

Nature of Alcohol Use

A large proportion (87%) of the population in England, ages 16 and above, report that they have consumed alcohol. This is slightly higher than the rates reported in the US, especially in the adolescent age group. While people with diabetes tend to drink less than their counterparts without diabetes, approximately one-third of adolescents with type 1 diabetes reported ongoing or sustained alcohol use [79, 80]. Although fewer individuals with type 1 diabetes drink alcohol, the potential and severity of harm associated with alcohol use are higher in people with diabetes than in the general population. In addition to the range of physical, psychological, and social harms experienced by the rest of the population, there are also specific effects of alcohol on diabetes and glycemic control.

Alcohol can have direct effects on blood glucose levels. The concern here is primarily from a hypoglycemia perspective. In the presence of alcohol, the steady stream of glucose secretion into the bloodstream by the liver is compromised because the liver devotes attention to removing the toxin from the body. This results in an imbalance between glucose and insulin in the body and can cause hypoglycemia. This can happen at several points in the course of alcohol consumption but often is more problematic as time passes. There is an increased likelihood of overnight and morning lows. Likewise, the possibility of a high during the consumption of alcohol, especially as part of a high-carbohydrate drink, is concerning as well. However, hypoglycemia has the potential to be far more dangerous immediately.

Alcohol may also have an indirect adverse effect on diabetes control. This can come in the form of lower levels of self-management (e.g., forgetting to inject insulin or monitor blood glucose) or engaging in risky behaviors, which in turn may have a negative impact on diabetes control, quality of life, and risk of depression [81].

Acute alcohol ingestion may induce an altered state of consciousness, resulting in reduced diabetes self-care. As with all substances, judgment is often impaired and the ability of the individual to manage this complex regimen is seriously jeopardized.

Screening for Alcohol Use

Late adolescence and young adulthood is a time of increasing responsibility and independence. New experiences are acquired, such as moving away from home, increased financial independence, and changes in peer groups and other relationships. Increased access to alcohol, with fewer familial restrictions or monitoring, is associated with increased alcohol consumption and alcohol-associated risk behaviors [82]. Considering these developmental and social changes, it is important to start screening early by asking probing questions about the availability of alcohol as well as the use in peer groups. Early education is essential and may lead to the prevention of serious problems that come with alcohol use.

Treatment Options

Our existing knowledge about what works in the treatment of psychological difficulties in children and young people with diabetes comes from several sources: intervention research with children and young people who are otherwise medically healthy, intervention research with adults with diabetes, and a small amount of work on diabetes-specific interventions. Much of these sources target depression and thus is the focus of this section. For more exhaustive reviews of family-based interventions and those focused on improving diabetes management in children and young people with diabetes, see the following resources [83, 84].

Many of the interventions that have been delivered to children and young people with type 1 diabetes have been family-based and have targeted promotion of diabetes management [85–88]. Typically, these interventions do not include children and young people with co-occurring depressive symptoms nor are depressive symptoms targeted in these treatments. Given the absence of an evidence base on effective treatments for children and young people with type 1 diabetes and co-occurring depressive symptoms, these children and young people are often treated with more general interventions. There is a substantial evidence base, however, for the efficacy of these general treatments. For example, Weisz and colleagues [89] conducted a meta-analysis on 35 studies and found an overall effect size of 0.34 in the reduction of depressive symptoms after treatment, compared with controls. Three-quarters of the studies included in that meta-analysis had cognitive change components (i.e., cognitive-behavioral therapy [CBT]) [90–92], and they collectively demonstrated a similar effect size of 0.35. Further, in the most comprehensive investigation of treatment options for adolescents with major depressive disorder, CBT was a necessary treatment component for the reduction of depressive symptoms [91]. The large-scale, NIMH-funded Treatment for Adolescents with Depression Study (TADS) examined three treatment arms (fluoxetine alone, CBT alone, fluoxetine + CBT) versus each other and placebo in 439 adolescents with major depressive disorder. The most effective treatment (effect size of 0.98 vs. placebo) was the combination treatment. When compared to the effect size of fluoxetine alone (0.68), the effect size difference due to CBT was very similar to what was found in the meta-analysis. However, long-term relapse data show lower rates in the participants treated with CBT, suggesting that the effects are consolidated later than medication effects and skills are learned in CBT that are utilized later [93].

CBT is an effective intervention for the reduction of depressive symptoms because of its grounding in cognitive and behavioral theories and treatment components that match those theories. Specifically, recent reviews by David-Ferdon and Kaslow [94] and prior work by Kazdin and Weisz [95] highlight the following components as primary targets of CBT: (1) increase participation in pleasant activities (that enhance mood), (2) increase and improve social interactions, (3) improve conflict resolution and social problem-solving skills, (4) reduce physiological tension or excessive affective arousal, and (5) identify and modify depressive thoughts and attributions. In other work conducted by Weisz and colleagues, they also point out that characteristics of effective interventions in the cognitive-behavioral framework often include homework to promote generalizability to real-world situations [96].

Presently, there are no studies that have tested whether CBT is effective in reducing depressive symptoms in children and young people with type 1 diabetes. Aspects of CBT show up in various treatments (e.g., Grey and colleagues work in coping skills training [87]), but it has not been the centerpiece of a treatment for children and young people with type 1 diabetes. There are, however, encouraging data in adults with diabetes that suggest CBT is likely to be effective in reducing depressive symptoms in adolescents with type 1 diabetes. Specifically, Lustman and colleagues [97] delivered CBT to adults with diabetes with major depressive disorder and found that the remission rate for the CBT group was 85%, nearly three times that of the control group. Further, a follow-up assessment of glycemic control showed a difference of 1.4% (9.5% in treated adults, 10.9% in controls). The authors hypothesized that the reduction of depressive symptoms led to better diabetes management, although they did not specifically test the mediating role of diabetes self-care behaviors. A more recent investigation of CBT by Amsberg and colleagues [98] showed similar results across reduced depressive symptoms and improved HbA1c values; however, they found a significant effect of CBT on self-care behavior. Specifically, they observed more frequent blood glucose monitoring in the participants receiving CBT early in treatment and that effect was maintained a year later. Considered together, in this small sample of studies on the effectiveness of CBT in adults with diabetes, CBT appears to reduce depressive symptoms and demonstrate benefits on diabetes self-management and glycemic outcomes. Further, these findings suggest support for the mediating role of self-care behaviors between depressive symptoms and glycemic control.

Summary and Conclusions

Children and young people with diabetes are charged with managing a disease that is chronic, unrelenting, and at times disruptive to daily life. Likewise, the parents and close family members of these children and young people are embedded in the life changes brought on by diabetes and many times are the individuals primarily responsible for its management. From this chapter, we hope it is clear that the emotional and behavioral health of the patients with diabetes, and their families, is critical to experience optimal health and quality of life outcomes. The diabetes clinician now has a broader set of tools to screen for those potentially disruptive emotional and behavioral problems and then move the family toward multiple options for treatment, whether that involves a focus on the individual or family, or both. Multiple cognitive-behavioral and family-based programs have been identified that strengthen the ability of individuals and families to manage diabetes effectively [87, 99, 100]. However, the critical first step is identification through screening, and this ideally raises the chances of better access to and more effectiveness of these evidence-based programs.

References

1. Cohen P, Cohen J, Kasen S, Velez CN, Hartmark C, Johnson J, et al. An epidemiological study of disorders in late childhood and adolescence–I. Age- and gender-specific prevalence. J Child Psychol Psychiatry. 1993;34(6):851–67. Epub 1993/09/01.
2. Reinherz HZ, Giaconia RM, Lefkowitz ES, Pakiz B, Frost AK. Prevalence of psychiatric disorders in a community population of older adolescents. J Am Acad Child Adolesc Psychiatry. 1993;32(2):369–77. Epub 1993/03/01.
3. Costello EJ, Angold A, Burns BJ, Stangl DK, Tweed DL, Erkanli A, et al. The great smoky mountains study of youth. Goals, design, methods, and the prevalence of DSM-III-R disorders. Arch Gen Psychiatry. 1996;53(12):1129–36. Epub 1996/12/01.
4. Lahey BB, Flagg EW, Bird HR, Schwab-Stone ME, Canino G, Dulcan MK, et al. The NIMH methods for the epidemiology of child and adolescent mental disorders (MECA) study: background and methodology. J Am Acad Child Adolesc Psychiatry. 1996;35(7):855–64. Epub 1996/07/01.
5. Lewinsohn PM, Rohde P, Seeley JR. Major depressive disorder in older adolescents: prevalence, risk factors, and clinical implications. Clin Psychol Rev. 1998;18(7):765–94. Epub 1998/11/25.
6. Canino G, Shrout PE, Rubio-Stipec M, Bird HR, Bravo M, Ramirez R, et al. The DSM-IV rates of child and adolescent disorders in Puerto Rico: prevalence, correlates, service use, and the effects of impairment. Arch Gen Psychiatry. 2004;61(1):85–93. Epub 2004/01/07.
7. Roberts RE, Roberts CR, Xing Y. Rates of DSM-IV psychiatric disorders among adolescents in a large metropolitan area. J Psychiatr Res. 2007;41(11):959–67. Epub 2006/11/17.
8. Brauner CB, Stephens CB. Estimating the prevalence of early childhood serious emotional/behavioral disorders: challenges and recommendations. Public Health Rep. 2006;121(3):303–10. Epub 2006/04/28.
9. Costello EJ, Egger H, Angold A. 10-year research update review: the epidemiology of child and adolescent psychiatric disorders: I. Methods and public health burden. J Am Acad Child Adolesc Psychiatry. 2005;44(10):972–86. Epub 2005/09/22.

10. Merikangas KR, He JP, Brody D, Fisher PW, Bourdon K, Koretz DS. Prevalence and treatment of mental disorders among US children in the 2001–2004 NHANES. Pediatrics. 2010;125(1):75–81. Epub 2009/12/17.
11. Merikangas KR, He JP, Burstein M, Swanson SA, Avenevoli S, Cui L, et al. Lifetime prevalence of mental disorders in US adolescents: results from the National Comorbidity Survey Replication–Adolescent Supplement (NCS-A). J Am Acad Child Adolesc Psychiatry. 2010; 49(10):980–9. Epub 2010/09/22.
12. Green H, McGinnity A, Meltzer H. Mental health of children and young people in Great Britian, 2004. Hampshire: Palgrave-Macmillan; 2005.
13. Meltzer H, Gatward R, Googman R, Ford T. The mental health of children and adolescents in Great Britian. London: Office of National Statistics; 2000.
14. Grey M, Whittemore R, Tamborlane W. Depression in type 1 diabetes in children: natural history and correlates. J Psychosom Res. 2002;53(4):907–11.
15. Hood KK, Huestis S, Maher A, Butler D, Volkening L, Laffel LM. Depressive symptoms in children and adolescents with type 1 diabetes: association with diabetes-specific characteristics. Diabetes Care. 2006;29(6):1389–91.
16. Kovacs M, Obrosky DS, Goldston D, Drash A. Major depressive disorder in youths with IDDM. A controlled prospective study of course and outcome. Diabetes Care. 1997;20(1):45–51.
17. Kokkonen J, Taanila A, Kokkonen E. Diabetes in adolescence: the effect of family and psychologic factors on metabolic control. Nord J Psychiatry. 1997;51:165–72.
18. Kovacs M, Goldston D, Obrosky DS, Bonar LK. Psychiatric disorders in youths with IDDM: rates and risk factors. Diabetes Care. 1997;20(1):36–44.
19. Stewart SM, Rao U, Emslie GJ, Klein D, White PC. Depressive symptoms predict hospitalization for adolescents with type 1 diabetes mellitus. Pediatrics. 2005;115(5):1315–9.
20. McGrady ME, Laffel L, Drotar D, Repaske D, Hood KK. Depressive symptoms and glycemic control in adolescents with type 1 diabetes: mediational role of blood glucose monitoring. Diabetes Care. 2009;32(5):804–6. Epub 2009/02/21.
21. Wysocki T, Iannotti R, Weissberg-Benchell J, Laffel L, Hood K, Anderson B, et al. Diabetes problem solving by youths with type 1 diabetes and their caregivers: measurement, validation, and longitudinal associations with glycemic control. J Pediatr Psychol. 2008;33(8):875–84. Epub 2008/03/19.
22. Grey M, Lipman T, Cameron ME, Thurber FW. Coping behaviors at diagnosis and in adjustment one year later in children with diabetes. Nurs Res. 1997;46(6):312–7.
23. Weissberg-Benchell J, Glasgow AM, Tynan WD, Wirtz P, Turek J, Ward J. Adolescent diabetes management and mismanagement. Diabetes Care. 1995;18(1):77–82.
24. Hood KK, Peterson CM, Rohan JM, Drotar D. Association between adherence and glycemic control in pediatric type 1 diabetes: a meta-analysis. Pediatrics. 2009;124(6):e1171–9.
25. Danne T, Mortensen HB, Hougaard P, Lynggaard H, Aanstoot HJ, Chiarelli F, et al. Persistent differences among centers over 3 years in glycemic control and hypoglycemia in a study of 3,805 children and adolescents with type 1 diabetes from the Hvidore Study Group. Diabetes Care. 2001;24(8):1342–7.
26. Svoren BM, Volkening LK, Butler DA, Moreland EC, Anderson BJ, Laffel LM. Temporal trends in the treatment of pediatric type 1 diabetes and impact on acute outcomes. J Pediatr. 2007;150(3):279–85. Epub 2007/02/20.
27. Mortensen HB, Hougaard P. Comparison of metabolic control in a cross-sectional study of 2,873 children and adolescents with IDDM from 18 countries. The Hvidore Study Group on Childhood Diabetes. Diabetes Care. 1997;20(5):714–20.
28. Forlenza GP, Rewers M. The epidemic of type 1 diabetes: what is it telling us? Curr Opin Endocrinol Diabetes Obes. 2011;18(4):248–51. Epub 2011/08/17.
29. Silverstein JH, Klingensmith G, Copeland K, Plotnick L, Kaufman F, Laffel L, et al. Care of children and adolescents with type 1 diabetes: a statement of the American Diabetes Association. Diabetes Care. 2005;28(1):186–212.
30. National Diabetes Data Group. Diabetes in America, 2nd edn. NIH Publication No. 95-1468. Bethesda: National Institutes of Health, National Institute of Diabetes and Digestive and Kidney Diseases; 1995.

31. American Diabetes Association. Economic costs of diabetes in the U.S. in 2007. Diabetes Care. 2008;31(3):596–615. Epub 2008/03/01.
32. Liese AD, D'Agostino Jr RB, Hamman RF, Kilgo PD, Lawrence JM, Liu LL, et al. The burden of diabetes mellitus among US youth: prevalence estimates from the SEARCH for diabetes in youth study. Pediatrics. 2006;118(4):1510–8.
33. Helgeson VS, Honcharuk E, Becker D, Escobar O, Siminerio L. A focus on blood glucose monitoring: relation to glycemic control and determinants of frequency. Pediatr Diabetes. 2011;12(1): 25–30. Epub 2010/06/05.
34. Diabetes Control and Complications Trial Research Group. Effect of intensive diabetes treatment on the development and progression of long-term complications in adolescents with insulin-dependent diabetes mellitus: diabetes control and complications trial. J Pediatr. 1994; 125(2):177–88.
35. Amstadter AB, Daughters SB, Macpherson L, Reynolds EK, Danielson CK, Wang F, et al. Genetic associations with performance on a behavioral measure of distress intolerance. J Psychiatr Res. 2012;46(1):87–94. Epub 2011/10/26.
36. La Greca AM, Auslander WF, Greco P, Spetter D, Fisher Jr EB, Santiago JV. I get by with a little help from my family and friends: adolescents' support for diabetes care. J Pediatr Psychol. 1995;20(4):449–76.
37. Anderson BJ, Holmbeck G, Iannotti RJ, McKay SV, Lochrie A, Volkening LK, et al. Dyadic measures of the parent–child relationship during the transition to adolescence and glycemic control in children with type 1 diabetes. Fam Syst Health. 2009;27(2):141–52.
38. Sullivan-Bolyai S, Deatrick J, Gruppuso P, Tamborlane W, Grey M. Mothers' experiences raising young children with type 1 diabetes. J Spec Pediatr Nurs. 2002;7(3):93–103. Epub 2002/09/19.
39. Anderson BJ, Ho J, Brackett J, Finkelstein D, Laffel L. Parental involvement in diabetes management tasks: relationships to blood glucose monitoring adherence and metabolic control in young adolescents with insulin-dependent diabetes mellitus. J Pediatr. 1997;130: 257–65.
40. Hood KK, Butler DA, Anderson BJ, Laffel LM. Updated and revised diabetes family conflict scale. Diabetes Care. 2007;30(7):1764–9.
41. Davis CL, Delamater AM, Shaw KH, La Greca AM, Eidson MS, Perez-Rodriguez JE, et al. Parenting styles, regimen adherence, and glycemic control in 4- to 10-year-old children with diabetes. J Pediatr Psychol. 2001;26(2):123–9.
42. Ellis DA, Podolski CL, Frey M, Naar-King S, Wang B, Moltz K. The role of parental monitoring in adolescent health outcomes: impact on regimen adherence in youth with type 1 diabetes. J Pediatr Psychol. 2007;32(8):907–17. Epub 2007/04/12.
43. Barnard KD, Lloyd CE, Skinner TC. Systematic literature review: quality of life associated with insulin pump use in type 1 diabetes. Diabet Med. 2007;24(6):607–17. Epub 2007/03/21.
44. World Health Organization. Mental health. Depression: what is depression. 2010. http://www.who.int/mental_health/management/depression/definition/en/. Accessed 16 Mar 2012.
45. Anderson RJ, Freedland KE, Clouse RE, Lustman PJ. The prevalence of comorbid depression in adults with diabetes: a meta-analysis. Diabetes Care. 2001;24(6):1069–78.
46. Reynolds KA, Helgeson VS. Children with diabetes compared to peers: depressed? Distressed? A meta-analytic review. Ann Behav Med. 2011;42(1):29–41. Epub 2011/03/30.
47. Anderson BJ, Edelstein S, Abramson NW, Katz LE, Yasuda PM, Lavietes SJ, et al. Depressive symptoms and quality of life in adolescents with type 2 diabetes: baseline data from the TODAY study. Diabetes Care. 2011;34(10):2205–7. Epub 2011/08/13.
48. Lawrence JM, Standiford DA, Loots B, Klingensmith GJ, Williams DE, Ruggiero A, et al. Prevalence and correlates of depressed mood among youth with diabetes: the SEARCH for diabetes in youth study. Pediatrics. 2006;117(4):1348–58. Epub 2006/04/06.
49. Delamater AM. Psychological care of children and adolescents with diabetes. Pediatr Diabetes. 2009;10 Suppl 12:175–84. Epub 2009/09/17.
50. Whooley MA, Avins AL, Miranda J, Browner WS. Case-finding instruments for depression. Two questions are as good as many. J Gen Intern Med. 1997;12(7):439–45. Epub 1997/07/01.
51. Arroll B, Khin N, Kerse N. Screening for depression in primary care with two verbally asked questions: cross sectional study. BMJ. 2003;327(7424):1144–6. Epub 2003/11/15.

52. Kovacs M. The Children's Depression Inventory (CDI): technical manual. North Tonawanda: Multi-Health Systems; 2003.
53. Radloff LS. The CES-D scale: a self-report depression scale for research in the general population. Appl Psychol Meas. 1977;1:385–401.
54. Dabelea D, Bell RA, D'Agostino Jr RB, Imperatore G, Johansen JM, Linder B, et al. Incidence of diabetes in youth in the United States. J Am Med Assoc. 2007;297(24):2716–24. Epub 2007/06/28.
55. Pouwer F, Tack CJ, Geelhoed-Duijvestijn PH, Bazelmans E, Beekman AT, Heine RJ, et al. Limited effect of screening for depression with written feedback in outpatients with diabetes mellitus: a randomised controlled trial. Diabetologia. 2011;54(4):741–8. Epub 2011/01/12.
56. Nouwen A, Lloyd CE, Pouwer F. Depression and type 2 diabetes over the lifespan: a meta-analysis. Response to Mezuk et al. Diabetes Care. 2009;32(5):e56; author reply e7. Epub 2009/05/02.
57. Kokoszka A, Pouwer F, Jodko A, Radzio R, Mucko P, Bienkowska J, et al. Serious diabetes-specific emotional problems in patients with type 2 diabetes who have different levels of comorbid depression: a Polish study from the European Depression in Diabetes (EDID) Research Consortium. Eur Psychiatry. 2009;24(7):425–30. Epub 2009/06/23.
58. Lewinsohn PM, Rohde P, Seeley JR, Klein DN, Gotlib IH. Natural course of adolescent major depressive disorder in a community sample: predictors of recurrence in young adults. Am J Psychiatry. 2000;157(10):1584–91.
59. Polonsky WH. Diabetes burnout: what to do when you can't take it anymore. New York: American Diabetes Association; 2000.
60. Polonsky WH, Anderson BJ, Lohrer PA, Welch G, Jacobson AM, Aponte JE, et al. Assessment of diabetes-related distress. Diabetes Care. 1995;18(6):754–60. Epub 1995/06/01.
61. Polonsky WH, Fisher L, Earles J, Dudl RJ, Lees J, Mullan J, et al. Assessing psychosocial distress in diabetes: development of the diabetes distress scale. Diabetes Care. 2005;28(3):626–31. Epub 2005/03/01.
62. Weissberg-Benchell J, Antisdel-Lomaglio J. Diabetes-specific emotional distress among adolescents: feasibility, reliability, and validity of the problem areas in diabetes-teen version. Pediatr Diabetes. 2011;12(4):341–4.
63. Hood KK, Butler DA, Volkening LK, Anderson BJ, Laffel LM. The Blood Glucose Monitoring Communication questionnaire: an instrument to measure affect specific to blood glucose monitoring. Diabetes Care. 2004;27(11):2610–5.
64. Markowitz JT, Volkening LK, Butler DA, Antisdel-Lomaglio J, Anderson BJ, Laffel LM. Re-examining a measure of diabetes-related burden in parents of young people with type 1 diabetes: the Problem Areas in Diabetes Survey – Parent Revised version (PAID-PR). Diabet Med. 2012;29:526–30.
65. Naar-King S, Idalski A, Ellis D, Frey M, Templin T, Cunningham PB, et al. Gender differences in adherence and metabolic control in urban youth with poorly controlled type 1 diabetes: the mediating role of mental health symptoms. J Pediatr Psychol. 2006;31(8):793–802. Epub 2005/12/03.
66. Herzer M, Hood KK. Anxiety symptoms in adolescents with type 1 diabetes: association with blood glucose monitoring and glycemic control. J Pediatr Psychol. 2010;35:415–25.
67. Dantzer C, Swendsen J, Maurice-Tison S, Salamon R. Anxiety and depression in juvenile diabetes: a critical review. Clin Psychol Rev. 2003;23(6):787–800.
68. Lloyd CE, Dyer PH, Barnett AH. Prevalence of symptoms of depression and anxiety in a diabetes clinic population. Diabet Med. 2000;17(3):198–202. Epub 2000/04/28.
69. Angold A, Costello EJ, Erkanli A. Comorbidity. J Child Psychol Psychiatry. 1999;40(1):57–87.
70. Spielberger CD. State-trait anxiety inventory for adults. Redwood City: Mind Garden; 1983.
71. The Diabetes Control and Complications Trial Research Group. The relationship of glycemic exposure (HbA1c) to the risk of development and progression of retinopathy in the diabetes control and complications trial. Diabetes. 1995;44(8):968–83.
72. Kamps JL, Roberts MC, Varela RE. Development of a new fear of hypoglycemia scale: preliminary results. J Pediatr Psychol. 2005;30(3):287–91. Epub 2005/03/24.
73. Green LB, Wysocki T, Reineck BM. Fear of hypoglycemia in children and adolescents with diabetes. J Pediatr Psychol. 1990;15(5):633–41. Epub 1990/10/01.

74. Barnard K, Thomas S, Royle P, Noyes K, Waugh N. Fear of hypoglycaemia in parents of young children with type 1 diabetes: a systematic review. BMC Pediatr. 2010;10:50. Epub 2010/07/17.
75. Patton SR, Dolan LM, Henry R, Powers SW. Parental fear of hypoglycemia: young children treated with continuous subcutaneous insulin infusion. Pediatr Diabetes. 2007;8(6):362–8. Epub 2007/11/27.
76. Cox DJ, Irvine A, Gonder-Frederick L, Nowacek G, Butterfield J. Fear of hypoglycemia: quantification, validation, and utilization. Diabetes Care. 1987;10(5):617–21. Epub 1987/09/01.
77. Gonder-Frederick LA, Fisher CD, Ritterband LM, Cox DJ, Hou L, DasGupta AA, et al. Predictors of fear of hypoglycemia in adolescents with type 1 diabetes and their parents. Pediatr Diabetes. 2006;7(4):215–22. Epub 2006/08/17.
78. Gonder-Frederick LA, Schmidt KM, Vajda KA, Greear ML, Singh H, Shepard JA, et al. Psychometric properties of the hypoglycemia fear survey-ii for adults with type 1 diabetes. Diabetes Care. 2011;34(4):801–6. Epub 2011/02/25.
79. Glasgow AM, Tynan D, Schwartz R, Hicks JM, Turek J, Driscol C, et al. Alcohol and drug use in teenagers with diabetes mellitus. J Adolesc Health. 1991;12(1):11–4. Epub 1991/01/01.
80. Martinez-Aguayo A, Araneda JC, Fernandez D, Gleisner A, Perez V, Codner E. Tobacco, alcohol, and illicit drug use in adolescents with diabetes mellitus. Pediatr Diabetes. 2007;8(5):265–71. Epub 2007/09/14.
81. Hislop AL, Fegan PG, Schlaeppi MJ, Duck M, Yeap BB. Prevalence and associations of psychological distress in young adults with type 1 diabetes. Diabet Med. 2008;25(1):91–6. Epub 2008/01/18.
82. Ramchandani N, Cantey-Kiser JM, Alter CA, Brink SJ, Yeager SD, Tamborlane WV, et al. Self-reported factors that affect glycemic control in college students with type 1 diabetes. Diabetes Educ. 2000;26(4):656–66. Epub 2001/01/05.
83. Jaser SS. Family interaction in pediatric diabetes. Curr Diab Rep. 2011;11(6):480–5. Epub 2011/08/20.
84. Hood KK, Rohan JM, Peterson CM, Drotar D. Interventions with adherence-promoting components in pediatric type 1 diabetes: meta-analysis of their impact on glycemic control. Diabetes Care. 2010;33(7):1658–64. Epub 2010/07/01.
85. Anderson BJ, Vangsness L, Connell A, Butler D, Goebel-Fabbri A, Laffel LM. Family conflict, adherence, and glycaemic control in youth with short duration type 1 diabetes. Diabet Med. 2002;19(8):635–42.
86. Wysocki T, Harris MA, Buckloh LM, Mertlich D, Lochrie AS, Taylor A, et al. Randomized, controlled trial of behavioral family systems therapy for diabetes: maintenance and generalization of effects on parent-adolescent communication. Behav Ther. 2008;39(1):33–46. Epub 2008/03/11.
87. Grey M, Boland EA, Davidson M, Li J, Tamborlane WV. Coping skills training for youth with diabetes mellitus has long-lasting effects on metabolic control and quality of life. J Pediatr. 2000;137(1):107–13.
88. Ellis DA, Frey MA, Naar-King S, Templin T, Cunningham P, Cakan N. Use of multisystemic therapy to improve regimen adherence among adolescents with type 1 diabetes in chronic poor metabolic control: a randomized controlled trial. Diabetes Care. 2005;28(7):1604–10. Epub 2005/06/29.
89. Weisz JR, McCarty CA, Valeri SM. Effects of psychotherapy for depression in children and adolescents: a meta-analysis. Psychol Bull. 2006;132(1):132–49.
90. Weisz JR. Psychotherapy for children and adolescents: evidence-based treatments and case examples. Cambridge: Cambridge University Press; 2004.
91. Treatment for Adolescents with Depression Study (TADS) Team. Fluoxetine, cognitive-behavioral therapy, and their combination for adolescents with depression. J Am Med Assoc. 2004; 292:807–20.
92. Reinecke MA, Ryan NE, DuBois DL. Cognitive-behavioral therapy of depression and depressive symptoms during adolescence: a review and meta-analysis. J Am Acad Child Adolesc Psychiatry. 1998;37(1):26–34.

93. Kennard BD, Silva SG, Tonev S, Rohde P, Hughes JL, Vitiello B, et al. Remission and recovery in the Treatment for Adolescents with Depression Study (TADS): acute and long-term outcomes. J Am Acad Child Adolesc Psychiatry. 2009;48(2):186–95. Epub 2009/01/08.
94. David-Ferdon C, Kaslow NJ. Evidence-based psychosocial treatments for child and adolescent depression. J Clin Child Adolesc Psychol. 2008;37(1):62–104. Epub 2008/04/30.
95. Kazdin AE, Weisz JR. Identifying and developing empirically supported child and adolescent treatments. J Consult Clin Psychol. 1998;66(1):19–36. Epub 1998/03/07.
96. Weisz JR, Doss AJ, Hawley KM. Youth psychotherapy outcome research: a review and critique of the evidence base. Annu Rev Psychol. 2005;56:337–63.
97. Lustman PJ, Griffith LS, Freedland KE, Kissel SS, Clouse RE. Cognitive behavior therapy for depression in type 2 diabetes mellitus. A randomized, controlled trial. Ann Intern Med. 1998;129(8):613–21. Epub 1998/10/24.
98. Amsberg S, Anderbro T, Wredling R, Lisspers J, Lins PE, Adamson U, et al. A cognitive behavior therapy-based intervention among poorly controlled adult type 1 diabetes patients – a randomized controlled trial. Patient Educ Couns. 2009;77:72–80. Epub 2009/03/20.
99. Wysocki T, Harris MA, Buckloh LM, Mertlich D, Lochrie AS, Taylor A, et al. Effects of behavioral family systems therapy for diabetes on adolescents' family relationships, treatment adherence, and metabolic control. J Pediatr Psychol. 2006;31(9):928–38.
100. Anderson BJ, Brackett J, Ho J, Laffel LM. An office-based intervention to maintain parent-adolescent teamwork in diabetes management. Impact on parent involvement, family conflict, and subsequent glycemic control. Diabetes Care. 1999;22(5):713–21.

Chapter 7
Depression in Older Adults with Diabetes: Measurement and Implications for Care

Elizabeth A. Beverly and Katie Weinger

Abstract Older patients with diabetes are at increased risk for multiple chronic conditions, including depression. Depression can impact on aspects of diabetes self-care including dietary self-management, exercise, and medication regimens and lead to poor glycemic control. Furthermore, depression is a major concern in older patients given that this population has the highest suicide rate of any age group. Thus, screening and treating depression in older diabetes patients is critical to improve health outcomes and reduce the risk of suicide. Despite increased awareness of comorbid depression and diabetes, diagnosis and treatment of depression in older diabetes patients remains a considerable challenge. Depression is frequently under-recognized and under-treated, with less than 25% of diabetes patients' depression successfully identified and treated in clinical practice. For older patients, depression may present with a variety of symptoms that vary from those observed in younger adults. Healthcare professionals have an important role in screening older diabetes patients at risk for depression and in identifying the number and severity of depressive symptoms. Several screening instruments have been developed that target depression in older patients or have been validated in this population; however, the validity of these instruments in older patients with diabetes requires further examination.

Keywords Diabetes • Older adults • Depression • Depression screening tools

---

E.A. Beverly, Ph.D. (✉) • K. Weinger, EdD, RN
Department of Clinical, Behavioral and Outcomes Research,
Joslin Diabetes Center,
Boston, MA, USA

Harvard Medical School, Boston, MA, USA
e-mail: elizabeth.beverly@joslin.harvard.edu; katie.weinger@joslin.harvard.edu

C.E. Lloyd et al. (eds.), *Screening for Depression and Other Psychological Problems in Diabetes*,
DOI 10.1007/978-0-85729-751-8_7, © Springer-Verlag London 2013

Introduction

Diabetes management in older patients presents unique challenges. Clinical (e.g., comorbidity, complications) and functional (e.g., impairment, disability) heterogeneity in the older population require special attention. Most diabetes patients have at least one comorbid condition [1] and as many as 40% have three or more distinct conditions [2]. Older diabetes patients are at greater risk for several geriatric syndromes, including depression, cognitive impairment, injurious falls, neuropathic pain, and urinary incontinence [3–10], with depression being one of the most serious geriatric syndromes impacting diabetes management. Comorbidities, such as depression, can have a deleterious effect on diabetes self-care [11–14], health status, and quality of life [15, 16]. Further, comorbidities that do not directly impact on self-care may pose competing demands, requiring substantial time, effort, and money to manage effectively [17–20]. Thus, understanding the impact of comorbidity on diabetes self-management is critical for improving diabetes treatment.

In this chapter, we review the current literature on depression, diabetes, and older adults. First, we discussed depression and diabetes in the older population, followed by barriers to diagnosis and treatment of depression. Next, we describe measurement tools for screening for depression in older patients. Finally, we discuss strategies and interventions that may be useful for clinicians to incorporate into practice.

Depression in Older Patients with Diabetes

Diabetes patients experience disproportionately high rates of depression, distress, and other social and emotional challenges [21–27]. An estimated 14–28% of older patients with diabetes have depression [28–31], which is approximately two to four times that of the general population aged 65 and older [32]. Depression can impact appropriate healthcare behaviors such as eating a healthy diet, exercise, and medication taking [11, 33, 34] and can lead to poor glycemic control [34]. Depression is also associated with the presence of serious complications (e.g., retinopathy, neuropathy, nephropathy, macrovascular complications of cardiovascular disease, hypertension, and sexual dysfunction [21, 35–38]), poor physical functioning [29], increased hospitalization, and mortality [39]. Further, depression in older patients is a major concern given that this population has the highest suicide rate of any age group [40, 41] (Facts Box). Thus, identifying and treating depression is critical to improve self-care and reduce the risk of suicide in older patients with diabetes (Clinical Box 1).

Facts Box

Older adults, depression, and suicide [41, 42]
Depression is one of the leading causes of suicide among older adults
Older adults account for 15.7% of all suicides
White men over the age of 85 are at the greatest risk for suicide of all age-gender-race groups
–84.4% of suicides in older adults were committed by men
Firearms were the most common means (71.9%) used for completing suicide

Clinical Box 1

Most common risk factors for suicide in older adults [43]
Recent death of a loved one
Social isolation and loneliness
Major change in social role (e.g., retirement)
Physical illness (e.g., uncontrollable pain, chronic illness)
Poor perceived health

Physical and psychosocial changes associated with aging can increase the risk for depression in older diabetes patients [44]. Decreases in muscle mass, aerobic capacity, visual and auditory acuity, bone strength, and joint flexibility contribute to physical, functional, and cognitive decline [44], which can lead to disability [45], impairment of activities of daily living [46, 47], poor perceived health [48], and lower quality of life [49]. Psychosocial changes, such as retirement, loss of family members and friends, loneliness, isolation, and fears about mortality, also can have a deleterious effect on diabetes and depression. Specifically, the helplessness and hopelessness commonly experienced by older patients can contribute to a negative cycle of exacerbating depressive symptoms, poor self-care, and worsening glycemic control [50]. Thus, timely diagnosis and effective treatment of comorbid depression in older patients is an essential component of quality diabetes care.

Barriers to Diagnosis of Depression

Diagnosis and treatment of comorbid depression in older patients is a considerable challenge in routine diabetes care. Depression is frequently under-recognized and under-treated [51–54], with less than 25% of diabetes patients' depression success-

Table 7.1 Typical and atypical depressive symptoms in older diabetes patients

Typical depressive symptoms	Atypical depressive symptoms [57]
Sad mood or affect	Denial or lack of sadness
Loss of pleasure or interest in activities	Unexplained somatic complaints
Tearfulness and crying spells	Hopelessness
Irritability[b]	Helplessness
Increased sense of worthlessness or guilt	Preoccupation with own mortality
Recurrent thoughts of suicide or death[c]	Anxiety and worries
Suicide threats or attempts[c]	Memory complaints
Loss of concentration[b]	Slowed speech and body movements
Decrease in recent memory[b]	Hyperactivity
Fatigue, loss of energy[b]	Seeing or hearing things that are not there
Pessimism	General lack of interest in personal care
Significant weight or appetite loss when not dieting, failure to gain age-appropriate weight	
Indecisiveness	
Social withdrawal or isolation	
Insomnia or hypersomnia[b]	
Psychomotor slowing[b]	
Psychomotor agitation	

[a]Depressed mood and 4 other symptoms for over 2 weeks may indicate major depression [58]
[b]Symptoms that may also reflect poorly controlled diabetes and/or hypoglycemia [59]
[c]Suicidal ideation should treated as a medical emergency and assessed immediately

fully identified and treated in clinical practice [55]. Furthermore, 75% of patients who recover from an episode of depression will suffer a relapse within 5 years [56]. For older patients, depression may present with a variety of cognitive, physical, affective, or attitudinal symptoms. Older patients' symptoms may also vary from typical depressive symptoms observed in younger adults [57] and thus may not meet the criteria from the American Psychiatric Association DSM-IV-TR [58]. Table 7.1 presents typical and atypical symptoms associated with depression in older patients. Importantly, physical and cognitive symptoms may overlap with poorly controlled diabetes, which can make the diagnosis of depression more difficult [59]. Further, if an older patient experiences depressed mood or loss of interest or pleasure in usual activities and at least four other depressive symptoms for a duration of at least 2 weeks, then major depression must be considered [60]. It should also be considered when these symptoms are accompanied by deterioration in glycemic control.

Other chronic health conditions associated with aging often contribute to the difficulties in identifying depression in older patients with diabetes [61] and increase the risk of suicide in the older population [62, 63]. Symptoms of depression (e.g., fatigue, changes in appetite) may overlap with other health conditions, such as thyroid disorders, sleep apnea, dementia, and alcohol or drug abuse, and polypharmacy [3, 64]. For example, depression and dementia share several overlapping symptoms including memory problems, psychomotor slowing, and changes in appetite and sleeping patterns (Table 7.2). However, differences in the time course and progression of symptoms can help distinguish between the two diagnoses [65]. Symptoms

Table 7.2 Typical presentation of symptoms of depression versus dementia [65]

Depression	Dementia
Onset of cognitive decline is rapid	Onset of cognitive decline is slow
Preoccupation about cognitive deficits	Lack of concern or denial about cognitive deficits
Difficulty concentrating	Difficulty with short-term memory
Knowledge of correct date, time, and location	Confusion and disorientation
Psychomotor slowing with rapid onset (language, body movements)	Impaired psychomotor skills with gradual onset (writing, speaking, facial masking)
Acute loss of interest or pleasure in activities	Gradual loss of interest or pleasure in activities
Acute changes in sleeping patterns	Gradual disruption of the sleep-wake cycle due to changes in the brain
Acute decrease in energy	Normal energy levels
Acute changes in appetite leading to weight loss or gain	Gradual changes in weight status over the course of months to years
Rapid onset of agitation, predominantly worse in the morning but may persist throughout the day	Gradual increase in agitation, predominantly worse in the late afternoon/evening (sundowning)
Suicidal ideation	No suicidal ideation

of sad mood or affect and the acute onset of cognitive decline, psychomotor slowing, loss of interest or pleasure in activities, and changes in sleeping patterns and appetite are likely to indicate depression. Whereas, a slow onset of cognitive decline, impairment of psychomotor skills, and gradual changes in appetite, sleeping patterns, and loss of interest or pleasure in activities are likely to represent dementia. In diabetes, hyperglycemia symptoms (e.g., loss of concentration, fatigue, hypersomnia, psychomotor slowing) and hypoglycemia symptoms (e.g., irritability, fatigue, decrease in recent memory) can mimic symptoms of depression (see Table 7.1). Thus, distinguishing between symptoms of depression and side effects of poorly controlled diabetes can be challenging. Clinicians should rule out these possibilities through physical examination, medical interview (including family history of depression), and laboratory investigations [65]. Failure to diagnose depression in older patients is serious because of the long-term, life-threatening risks for complications [21, 35–38], functional disability, hospitalization, and mortality [39].

Patient and clinician barriers can also contribute to the difficulty diagnosing depression in older patients with diabetes (Table 7.3). Older patients and their family members may attach stigma to depression and consequently disagree with a clinician's diagnosis of depression [66]. Furthermore, patients may be reluctant to communicate symptoms of depression due to treatment-related concerns (e.g., financial, medication) [67, 68], prioritization of other health conditions [20], or lack of a support system [69]. Older patients may also have difficulty recognizing the symptoms of depression because they often present atypically [57]. Similarly, clinicians may struggle with the identification of depression because they lack the knowledge of atypical depression symptoms [57, 69] and/or psychological expertise to diagnose patients with depression [70, 71]. At the

Table 7.3 Patient and provider barriers to diagnosing depression [57, 67–69, 71–73]

Patient barriers	Clinician barriers
Stigma related to mental illness	Lack of knowledge of atypical depression symptoms in older patients
Family members' stigma related to mental illness	Perceived lack of psychological expertise
Lack of a support system	Fear of compromising patient confidentiality
Financial concerns for treatment (insurance coverage)	Stigma related to mental illness
Limited availability of mental health resources	Ageism or belief that depression is a normal part of the aging process
Other chronic health conditions take priority in self-care	Unwillingness to listen to patients' struggles
Difficulty recognizing the symptoms of depression	Other chronic health conditions take priority during a short medical visit
Reluctance to discuss depression symptoms with provider	Belief that overlapping symptoms from other chronic conditions explain depression symptoms
Attributing depressive symptoms to another health condition	Belief that antidepressants will interfere with treatment of other health conditions or interact with other medications
Belief that antidepressants are addictive	Lack of knowledge of proper depression screening tools

same time, other chronic health conditions may take precedence during an already time-constrained medical visit. Lastly, clinicians may harbor stigma related to mental illness or believe that depression is a normal part of the aging process [67]. Thus, underdiagnosis of depression in older patients with diabetes is a serious healthcare challenge.

Instruments for Screening for Depression in Older Patients

Diabetes care guidelines recommend older patients be screened for depression using a standardized screening tool during the initial evaluation and when there is deterioration in glycemic control and/or unexplained decline in health status [3, 74]. Screening is used primarily to identify patients at high risk for depression. Appropriate instruments are characterized by brief administration and straightforward scoring systems that provide an estimate of the number and severity of depressive symptoms [75]. Screening instruments that have been developed to target depression in older patients or have been validated in this population include the Geriatric Depression Scale (GDS) [76, 77], Depressive Symptom Assessment for Older Adults (DSA) [78], the Detection of Depression in the Elderly Scale (DDES) [79, 80], Cornell Scale for Depression in Dementia (CSDD) [81, 82], Center for Epidemiologic

Table 7.4 Summary of depression screening tools for older patients

Screening tool	Items	Rating	Time to complete	Cost
Geriatric Depression Scale (GDS)	30	Self-administered	10–15 min	None
Geriatric Depression Scale 15 (GDS-15)	15	Self-administered	5–10 min	None
Depressive Symptom Assessment for Older Adults (DSA)	27	Clinician interviewer	10–30 min	None
Detection of Depression in the Elderly Scale (DDES)	25	Self-administered	10–15 min	None
Cornell Scale for Depression in Dementia (CSDD)	19	Clinician interviewer	10 min with patient; 20 min with informant	None
Center for Epidemiologic Studies Depression Scale (CES-D)	20	Self-administered	5–10 min	None
Beck Depression Inventory (BDI-II)	21	Self-administered	20 min	$75 for manual and 25 record forms. *Additional forms are $40 for 25 or $145 for 100
World Health Organization 5-item Well-Being Index (WHO-5)	5	Self-administered	5 min	None
Patient Health Questionnaire-9 (PHQ-9)	9	Self-administered	1–2 min	None

Studies Depression Scale (CES-D) [83], the Beck Depression Inventory (BDI) [84], the World Health Organization 5-item Well-Being Index (WHO-5) [85–87], and the Patient Health Questionnaire-9 (PHQ-9) [88]. Below we describe these measurement tools in terms of screening for depression in older patients (Table 7.4).

Geriatric Depression Scale (GDS)

The Geriatric Depression Scale (GDS) is one of the most widely used screening tools for depression among older adults. The GDS contains 30 questions, each requiring a yes/no response [76, 77]. The scale demonstrates good reliability [89], good convergent validity with other depression scales [76, 90], and adequate sensitivity [91]. Furthermore, the GDS compares favorably with diagnostic interviews for major depression [92] but less favorably with criteria for less severe depression

[93]. Overall, the GDS is useful in screening for depression in older patients; however, it is a lengthy instrument. For this reason, shorter versions of the GDS have been developed: the GDS-15 [94], GDS-12R [95], GDS-10 [96], GDS-5 [97], GDS-4 [96], and the GDS one-item version [98]. Most of these shortened versions demonstrate high sensitivity (ranging from 88.9% to 100%) yet variable specificity (ranging from 18.9% to 75.7%), with the exception of the GDS one-item version (sensitivity 14.8%, specificity 97.9%) [99].

While the GDS is a widely used instrument for older patients, it has several limitations. First, the GDS is self-rated and requires patients to fill out a questionnaire, which may be challenging for older adults with literacy, visual, or mobility impairments [78, 100–103]. Second, the yes/no response format does not provide in-depth information, which could be useful for tailoring treatments to older patients. Third, the GDS does not contain a question about suicide despite this population having the highest suicide rate of any age group [104, 105]. The GDS also does not include questions about appetite or sleep changes because these symptoms often overlap with normal age-related changes [104, 105]. Furthermore, although the GDS is widely used for screening for depression in older patients, the validity of this measure in older patients with diabetes has not been examined. Importantly, the GDS is not validated in older populations with moderate to severe dementia [100, 102, 103].

Depressive Symptom Assessment for Older Adults (DSA)

The Depressive Symptom Assessment for Older Adults (DSA) provides a comprehensive measure of depression for older patients regardless of cognitive status. The DSA is a 27-item interviewer-rated instrument based on the Hamilton Rating Scale for Depression [106], an interviewer-rated scale for adults of all ages, and the Dementia Mood Assessment Scale, an observer-rated scale for older adults with dementia [107]. For each of the 27 items, the interviewer evaluates the affect, speech, and behavior of the older patient in addition to information obtained from medical records and caregivers [78]. The total score ranges from 0 to 81, with each item ranging from 0 to 3 (0 = none, 1 = mild, 2 = moderate, 3 = severe). The DSA has six subscales: (1) melancholic behavior, (2) disagreeable behavior, (3) anxiety, (4) sleep impairment, (5) appetite impairment, and (6) lack of meaning in life. These subscales enable clinicians to identify manifestations of depression that could be missed and to provide targeted treatment for depressive symptoms [78]. In general, the DSA demonstrates good content validity and is a comprehensive, interviewer-rated method to assess depression in older patients regardless of their cognitive status. Drawbacks of the DSA include the lengthy administration (10–30 min), the degree of clinical skill required to administer the assessment, and the fact that this assessment has not yet been validated in older patients with diabetes.

Detection of Depression in the Elderly Scale (DDES)

The Detection of Depression in the Elderly Scale (DDES) is a 25-item instrument designed specifically to detect major depression in older patients aged 65 and older in primary care [80]. The DDES demonstrates appropriate reliability indices (test-retest reliability = 0.858; inter-rater reliability = 0.908) and good internal consistency (Cronbach's alpha = 0.79) [80]. Further, the DDES has high sensitivity (90.4%) and moderate specificity (74.8%) [80]. Compared to the GDS, the DDES may be a more sensitive tool for the detection of depression in primary care, with fewer false negatives for major depression [79]. Thus, the DDES is a clinically useful instrument for the detection of major depression in older patients aged 65 and older in a primary care setting; however, this scale is relatively new and has not been validated in older patients with diabetes.

Cornell Scale for Depression in Dementia (CSDD)

The Cornell Scale for Depression in Dementia (CSDD) is a 19-item comprehensive interview specifically developed to assess signs and symptoms of major depression in patients with dementia [81, 82]. Signs and symptoms of depression are grouped into five areas: (1) mood (e.g., sadness, anxiety, irritability), (2) behavioral disturbances (e.g., agitation, psychomotor slowing), (3) physical symptoms (e.g., loss of appetite, weight loss), (4) cyclic functioning (e.g., sleep disturbances, diurnal mood variation), and (5) ideational aspects of depression (e.g., suicidal thoughts, pessimism, low self-esteem) [108]. The interview elicits information from an informant (e.g., family member, caregiver) and the patient; administration takes approximately 20 min with the informant and 10 min with the patient. Each item is rated from 0 to 2 (0 = absent, 1 = mild or intermittent, 2 = severe). Items are summed to yield a total score. A score above 10 indicates probable major depression, and a score above 18 indicates definite major depression [81]. In our view, the CSDD is the best validated scale to assess depressive symptoms in patients with dementia [109].

Center for Epidemiologic Studies Depression Scale (CES-D)

The Center for Epidemiologic Studies Depression Scale (CES-D) is one of the most widely used self-report depression instruments and has become a standard measure of depression symptoms in older patients [83]. The CES-D is a 20-item index that measures depressive feelings and behaviors during the past week using a four-response format (0 = "rarely or none of the time (<1 day)"; 1 = "some or a little of the time (1–2 days)"; 3 = "occasionally or a moderate amount of the time (3–4 days)"; 4 = "most or all of the time (5–7 days)"). The 20 items comprise six scales reflecting major dimensions of depression: (1) depressed mood, (2) feelings of guilt and worthlessness, (3) feelings of helplessness and hopelessness, (4) psychomotor retardation, (5) loss of appetite, and (6) sleep disturbance [83]. A score of 16 or higher is the established cutoff point for high depressive symptoms on this scale [83]. In a subset of the population aged 65 years and older, the CES-D showed good internal consistency (Cronbach's alpha > 0.85) and test-retest correlations remained >0.40 [83]. However, pretests of the CES-D in an older sample revealed that the original 20-item version may be taxing for this population and increase the likelihood of false positives [110].

Thus, a brief, 11-item version of the CES-D was developed for screening for depression in older patients [111]. The 11-item scale is highly correlated with the 20-item version (Pearson $r=0.95$, $n=2339$) [111]. The 11-item CES-D contains a three response format (0 = "hardly ever or never"; 1 = "some of the time"; 2 = "much or most of the time") for each item. Six symptoms scored at a 1 or 2 level, or eight symptoms scored at a 1 level correspond to the 16 or higher cutoff score from the original CES-D [112]. Importantly, the 20-item and 11-item CES-D scales are not DSM-based measures of depression and should not be used as clinical diagnostic tools.

Beck Depression Inventory (BDI)

The Beck Depression Inventory (BDI, BDI-II) is a 21-item self-report instrument for measuring the severity of depression [113, 114] (see Chap. 4 for more details). The items assess various symptoms of depression including hopelessness and irritability, cognitions such as guilt or feelings of being punished, and physical symptoms such as fatigue and weight loss/gain. The BDI-II uses a four-response format, with each answer scored on a scale of 0–3 (note: two items include seven options to indicate an increase or decrease of appetite and sleep). The cutoffs scores are as follows: 0–13: minimal depression, 14–19: mild depression, 20–28: moderate depression, and 29–63: severe depression [114].

In a sample of older community-dwelling adults ranging in age from 50 to 90 years, the BDI-II demonstrated strong psychometric properties, including good internal consistency ($\alpha=0.86$), good internal reliability ($\alpha=0.90$), and solid convergent and discriminant validity via correlations with other measures, including the CES-D, the Coolidge Axis II Inventory (CATI) Depression subscale, and the Perceived Stress Scale (PSS) [115]. In a second sample of 64 older women recruited from independent living facilities, the BDI-II was positively correlated with the GDS ($r=0.71$), and both the BDI-II and GDS demonstrated good internal consistency ($r=0.85$ and 0.84, respectively) [116]. Thus, the BDI-II holds promise as a valuable assessment tool for measuring depression in older adults.

In one study of diabetes patients, the BDI-II effectively differentiated depressed patients from nondepressed patients, with a cutoff score of >12 yielding sensitivity and specificity values of 0.90 and 0.84 and a cutoff score of >16 yielding sensitivity and specificity values of 0.73 and 0.93 [117]. Thus, it appears that the BDI-II is an effective screening tool for major depression in patients with diabetes; however, the validity of this measure in older patients with diabetes has not been examined.

World Health Organization 5-Item Well-Being Index (WHO-5)

The World Health Organization 5-Item Well-Being Index (WHO-5) is a 5-item, one-dimensional measure of emotional well-being (see Chap. 4 for more details). Each item is positively worded indicating the degree to which positive feelings were present or absent in the last 2 weeks on a 6-point Likert scale ranging from 0 (not present) to 5 (constantly present) [118]. Scores are summed yielding a total score, which is then standardized to a 100-point scale. A higher score represents better emotional well-being; a cutoff score of 13 or less can be used to define depression [85]. The WHO-5 demonstrates high sensitivity as a screening tool for depression in adults with diabetes [85, 119] and with older adults [120–122]. In a Japanese sample of older adults aged 70 years and older, the WHO-5 successfully discriminated older patients with suicidal ideation, and when combined with the Scale of Perceived Social Support (PSS) [123, 124], more effectively identified older adults with suicidal ideation than the WHO-5 alone (sensitivity = 87%, specificity = 75%, negative predictive value = 99%, and positive predictive value = 10%) [119]. In sum, the WHO-5 is a short screening instrument that can be completed in less than 5 min and should be used more widely for depression screening in older patients [85]. Further, the WHO-5 has predictive utility in detecting suicidal ideation in older adults, which is particularly relevant given that older adults have the highest rate of suicide.

Patient Health Questionnaire-9 (PHQ-9)

The Patient Health Questionnaire-9 (PHQ-9) is a 9-item depression scale derived from the full Patient Health Questionnaire [88] (see Chap. 4). This multipurpose instrument is useful for screening, diagnosing, monitoring, and measuring severity of depression. PHQ-9 scores of 5, 10, 15, and 20 correspond to mild, moderate, moderately severe, and severe depression [88]. In a study of older adults aged 65 years and older (mean = 78), the PHQ-9 performed comparably with the GDS-15 for identifying major depression in a primary care setting [125]. Furthermore, this questionnaire has been administered to older patients where it was found to be sensitive to changes in depression symptom severity when compared to the Symptom Checklist-20, a standardized depression severity measure [126]. Further, the PHQ-9 has been validated in patients with diabetes where a cutoff score of 12 resulted in a sensitivity of 75.7% and a specificity of 80.0% [127]. Thus, the PHQ-9 is an effective screening instrument for major depression in older patients and patients with diabetes. In summary, the PHQ-9 is brief and can be easily administered in clinical practice. This tool is useful for assisting clinicians in diagnosing depression as well as selecting and monitoring treatment.

Implications for Clinicians

Treatment of depression in the older population must consider nonglycemic risk factors that contribute to standard microvascular and macrovascular complications as well as common geriatric syndromes. Older patients with diabetes and depression are at increased risk of multiple chronic conditions and poor physical functioning [29]. Both microvascular and macrovascular complications disproportionately affect older patients with diabetes and depression [128–133] and are a major cause of excess mortality [134–138]. Specifically, depression is associated with the presence of retinopathy, cardiovascular disease, neuropathy, nephropathy, hypertension, and sexual dysfunction [21, 35–38]. Further, high rates of comorbid illness may require older adults to take multiple medications, including antidepressants, which can lead to drug side effects and drug-drug and drug-disease interactions [3]. Thus, a multifactorial approach to screening and treating depression in older patients is necessary. The overall goals of diabetes treatment should aim towards optimizing function and reducing the burden of morbidity and mortality in the older segment of the population.

Diabetes care guidelines recommend psychosocial screening assessments be included as part of ongoing diabetes management [74]. A psychosocial screening [74] should include assessments of, but not limited to, depression [76, 77, 83, 84, 139, 140], diabetes attitudes [141], diabetes-related quality of life [142, 143], diabetes-related distress [25, 144], expectations for medical management and outcomes, general affect and mood [140], psychiatric history [145–147], and resources (e.g., financial, social) [148]. Incorporating psychosocial screening assessments in standard medical visits may improve the identification and treatment of depression in older adults. Further, brief, effective screening tools may aid clinicians in recognizing depression during a medical visit. Asking two simple questions such as "during the past month, have you felt down, depressed, or hopeless?" and "during the past month, have you lost interest or pleasure in doing things?" can be as successful as surveys when screening for depression [149].

Lastly, a vital component of diabetes care is individualization. Older patients vary both clinically and functionally. As emphasized in clinical care guidelines [3, 74], no two older patients are alike, and every patient needs an individualized diabetes treatment plan. Individualized care should take into account health status, life expectancy, personalized goals for treatment, willingness and ability to comply with proposed treatment regimen, financial resources, and home care situation [132]. What works for one patient may not be the best course of treatment for another. For some patients, maintaining functional independence in activities of daily living and minimizing the psychological burden of diabetes may take precedence over aggressive medical management, while others may prefer intensive treatment and long-term preventive care strategies [150]. Clinicians should respect older patients' wants, needs, and preferences while providing the proper education and support to assist older patients in making informed decisions about their care. Diabetes care is a continuous process. Older patients and their clinicians should engage in ongoing discussions about what care is best for them and why (Clinical Box 2). Discussing perceived challenges to depression and diabetes may provide a systematic way to include older participants in the evaluation and treatment process, thereby enhancing therapeutic alliance. Over time, the treatment process should become an open dialogue continually redefining and attending to the ever-changing needs of older patients.

Clinical Box 2

How to approach the topic of depression with older people with diabetes	
Help the patient understand depression	Patients may have different views and opinions about depression. For example, older patients may think depression is a normal part of aging. Clinicians may need to explain that depression is medical condition that can complicate diabetes self-management. Further, clinicians may need to explain treatment options and mental health resources
Speak in easily understood language and terminology	Communicating openly and effectively with patients about depression requires talking about it in terms that are comfortable for both the clinician and patient. Using terminology and examples/analogies that are familiar to the patient can be helpful
Ask open-ended questions	Open-ended questions allow patients to verbalize feelings in their own words and provide health information that is important to them. Sample questions include: "How are you feeling?" "What problems are you having?" "Have you noticed any changes since you started taking the antidepressant?"
Be a good, active listener	Clinicians may hold preconceived notions about what a patient means or says during a medical visit. Active listening requires clinicians to focus on what the patient is actually saying. Reflecting or repeating statements back to the patient and summarizing the conversation are helpful strategies to demonstrate that the clinician has been listening and understands what the patient means.
Be supportive	Coping with the challenges of depression and its symptoms can be difficult. Clinicians should be empathetic to patients' struggles rather than judgmental. Remembering to ask the patient how he/she feels, acknowledging the complexity of diabetes self-care, and scheduling more frequent follow-up visits are strategies that support your patient
Recognize that this is an ongoing process	Some older patients may be unwilling to accept a diagnosis of depression. Diagnosing and treating depression is an ongoing process. Open dialogue is necessary to continually redefine and attend to the ever-changing needs of older patients (e.g., new symptoms, comorbid conditions, medications) and thus individualize treatment prescriptions and recommendations

In summary, contemporary issues, such as clinical and functional heterogeneity, challenge the health community to provide comprehensive care to older patients with diabetes and depression. Clinicians should be cognizant of older patients' comorbid conditions, like depression, and their impact on diabetes management. Further, the research community should more aggressively address the psychosocial and emotional needs of older patients. As the prevalence of diabetes burgeons among our aging population, the healthcare community should strengthen clinical guidelines to maximize successful care and, ultimately, improve both the length and quality of life experienced by older patients with diabetes and depression.

Conclusion

Older patients with diabetes are at increased risk for geriatric syndromes, including depression. Depression impacts older patients' ability to carry out self-care behaviors and follow through with treatment recommendations. This inability may limit the success of treatment regimens designed to improve glycemic control and prevent diabetes complications. We have described several clinical assessment tools used to identify depression in older patients with diabetes, and have offered strategies that clinicians can employ to improve the identification and treatment of depression in their clinical practice. Clinicians are well positioned to recognize the cues of older adults struggling to manage their diabetes amidst depression and/or other health conditions.

References

1. Druss BG, Marcus SC, Olfson M, Tanielian T, Elinson L, Pincus HA. Comparing the national economic burden of five chronic conditions. Health Aff (Millwood). 2001;20(6):233–41.
2. Wolff JL, Starfield B, Anderson G. Prevalence, expenditures, and complications of multiple chronic conditions in the elderly. Arch Intern Med. 2002;162(20):2269–76.
3. Brown AF, Mangione CM, Saliba D, Sarkisian CA. Guidelines for improving the care of the older person with diabetes mellitus. J Am Geriatr Soc. 2003;51(5 Suppl Guidelines):S265–80.
4. Guideline for the prevention of falls in older persons. American Geriatrics Society, British Geriatrics Society, and American Academy of Orthopaedic Surgeons Panel on Falls Prevention. J Am Geriatr Soc. 2001;49(5):664–72.
5. Shekelle PG, MacLean CH, Morton SC, Wenger NS. Assessing care of vulnerable elders: methods for developing quality indicators. Ann Intern Med. 2001;135(8 Pt 2):647–52.
6. Ueda T, Tamaki M, Kageyama S, Yoshimura N, Yoshida O. Urinary incontinence among community-dwelling people aged 40 years or older in Japan: prevalence, risk factors, knowledge and self-perception. Int J Urol. 2000;7(3):95–103.
7. Cummings SR, Nevitt MC, Browner WS, Stone K, Fox KM, Ensrud KE, et al. Risk factors for hip fracture in white women. Study of Osteoporotic Fractures Research Group. N Engl J Med. 1995;332(12):767–73.
8. Dealberto MJ, Seeman T, McAvay GJ, Berkman L. Factors related to current and subsequent psychotropic drug use in an elderly cohort. J Clin Epidemiol. 1997;50(3):357–64.

9. Newman SC, Hassan AI. Antidepressant use in the elderly population in Canada: results from a national survey. J Gerontol A Biol Sci Med Sci. 1999;54(10):M527–30.
10. Piven ML. Detection of depression in the cognitively intact older adult protocol. J Gerontol Nurs. 2001;27(6):8–14.
11. Ciechanowski PS, Katon WJ, Russo JE. Depression and diabetes: impact of depressive symptoms on adherence, function, and costs. Arch Intern Med. 2000;160(21):3278–85.
12. Schoenberg NE, Drungle SC. Barriers to non-insulin dependent diabetes mellitus (NIDDM) self-care practices among older women. J Aging Health. 2001;13(4):443–66.
13. Krein SL, Heisler M, Piette JD, Makki F, Kerr EA. The effect of chronic pain on diabetes patients' self-management. Diabetes Care. 2005;28(1):65–70.
14. Kerr EA, Heisler M, Krein SL, Kabeto M, Langa KM, Weir D, et al. Beyond comorbidity counts: how do comorbidity type and severity influence diabetes patients' treatment priorities and self-management? J Gen Intern Med. 2007;22(12):1635–40.
15. Glasgow RE, Ruggiero L, Eakin EG, Dryfoos J, Chobanian L. Quality of life and associated characteristics in a large national sample of adults with diabetes. Diabetes Care. 1997;20(4):562–7.
16. Wray LA, Ofstedal MB, Langa KM, Blaum CS. The effect of diabetes on disability in middle-aged and older adults. J Gerontol A Biol Sci Med Sci. 2005;60(9):1206–11.
17. Jaen CR, Stange KC, Nutting PA. Competing demands of primary care: a model for the delivery of clinical preventive services. J Fam Pract. 1994;38(2):166–71.
18. Chernof BA, Sherman SE, Lanto AB, Lee ML, Yano EM, Rubenstein LV. Health habit counseling amidst competing demands: effects of patient health habits and visit characteristics. Med Care. 1999;37(8):738–47.
19. Bayliss EA, Steiner JF, Fernald DH, Crane LA, Main DS. Descriptions of barriers to self-care by persons with comorbid chronic diseases. Ann Fam Med. 2003;1(1):15–21.
20. Beverly EA, Wray LA, Chiu CJ, Weinger K. Perceived challenges and priorities in co-morbidity management of older patients with Type 2 diabetes. Diabet Med. 2011;28(7):781–4.
21. de Groot M, Anderson R, Freedland KE, Clouse RE, Lustman PJ. Association of depression and diabetes complications: a meta-analysis. Psychosom Med. 2001;63(4):619–30.
22. Anderson RJ, Freedland KE, Clouse RE, Lustman PJ. The prevalence of comorbid depression in adults with diabetes: a meta-analysis. Diabetes Care. 2001;24(6):1069–78.
23. Lloyd CE, Dyer PH, Barnett AH. Prevalence of symptoms of depression and anxiety in a diabetes clinic population. Diabet Med. 2000;17(3):198–202.
24. Weinger K, Jacobson AM. Psychosocial and quality of life correlates of glycemic control during intensive treatment of type 1 diabetes. Patient Educ Couns. 2001;42(2):123–31.
25. Welch GW, Jacobson AM, Polonsky WH. The problem areas in diabetes scale. An evaluation of its clinical utility. Diabetes Care. 1997;20(5):760–6.
26. Gonzalez JS, Peyrot M, McCarl LA, Collins EM, Serpa L, Mimiaga MJ, et al. Depression and diabetes treatment nonadherence: a meta-analysis. Diabetes Care. 2008;31(12):2398–403.
27. Rubin RR, Peyrot M, Siminerio LM. Health care and patient-reported outcomes: results of the cross-national Diabetes Attitudes, Wishes and Needs (DAWN) study. Diabetes Care. 2006; 29(6):1249–55.
28. Kessler RC, Berglund P, Demler O, Jin R, Koretz D, Merikangas KR, et al. The epidemiology of major depressive disorder: results from the National Comorbidity Survey Replication (NCS-R). JAMA. 2003;289(23):3095–105.
29. Bell RA, Smith SL, Arcury TA, Snively BM, Stafford JM, Quandt SA. Prevalence and correlates of depressive symptoms among rural older African Americans, Native Americans, and whites with diabetes. Diabetes Care. 2005;28(4):823–9.
30. Bruce DG, Casey GP, Grange V, Clarnette RC, Almeida OP, Foster JK, et al. Cognitive impairment, physical disability and depressive symptoms in older diabetic patients: the Fremantle Cognition in Diabetes Study. Diabetes Res Clin Pract. 2003;61(1):59–67.
31. Chou KL, Chi I. Prevalence of depression among elderly Chinese with diabetes. Int J Geriatr Psychiatry. 2005;20(6):570–5.
32. Current Depression Among Adults – United States, 2006–2008. Centers for Disease Control and Prevention, U.S. Department of Health & Human Services, Atlanta; 2010.

33. Lin EH, Katon W, Von Korff M, Rutter C, Simon GE, Oliver M, et al. Relationship of depression and diabetes self-care, medication adherence, and preventive care. Diabetes Care. 2004; 27(9):2154–60.
34. Lustman PJ, Anderson RJ, Freedland KE, de Groot M, Carney RM, Clouse RE. Depression and poor glycemic control: a meta-analytic review of the literature. Diabetes Care. 2000; 23(7):934–42.
35. Kovacs M, Mukerji P, Drash A, Iyengar S. Biomedical and psychiatric risk factors for retinopathy among children with IDDM. Diabetes Care. 1995;18(12):1592–9.
36. Lustman PJ, Griffith LS, Gavard JA, Clouse RE. Depression in adults with diabetes. Diabetes Care. 1992;15(11):1631–9.
37. Jacobson AM. The psychological care of patients with insulin-dependent diabetes mellitus. N Engl J Med. 1996;334(19):1249–53.
38. Cohen HW, Gibson G, Alderman MH. Excess risk of myocardial infarction in patients treated with antidepressant medications: association with use of tricyclic agents. Am J Med. 2000;108(1):2–8.
39. Rosenthal MJ, Fajardo M, Gilmore S, Morley JE, Naliboff BD. Hospitalization and mortality of diabetes in older adults. A 3-year prospective study. Diabetes Care. 1998;21(2):231–5.
40. Centers for Disease Control and Prevention. Web-based Injury Statistics Query and Reporting System (WISQARS) [Online]. National Center for Injury Prevention and Control, Centers for Disease Control and Prevention (producer); 2007. http://www.cdc.gov/injury/wisqars/index.html. Accessed 19 Dec. 2012.
41. National Institute of Mental Health. Suicide in the U.S.: Statistics and Prevention (NIH Publication No. 06-4594). Retrieved from National Institute of Mental Health; 2010. http://www.nimh.nih.gov/health/publications/suicide-in-the-us-statistics-and-prevention/index.shtml.
42. National Center for Injury Prevention and Control. Web-based Injury Statistics Query and Reporting System (WISQARS). Atlanta: Centers for Disease Control and Prevention; 2010.
43. American Association of Suicidology. Elderly suicide fact sheet. Washington, DC: American Association of Suicidology; 2009.
44. Trief PM. Depression in elderly diabetes patients. Diabetes Spectr. 2007;20(2):71–5.
45. Egede LE. Diabetes, major depression, and functional disability among U.S. adults. Diabetes Care. 2004;27(2):421–8.
46. Gregg EW, Beckles GL, Williamson DF, Leveille SG, Langlois JA, Engelgau MM, et al. Diabetes and physical disability among older U.S. adults. Diabetes Care. 2000;23(9): 1272–7.
47. Volpato S, Blaum C, Resnick H, Ferrucci L, Fried LP, Guralnik JM. Comorbidities and impairments explaining the association between diabetes and lower extremity disability: the Women's Health and Aging Study. Diabetes Care. 2002;25(4):678–83.
48. Black SA. Increased health burden associated with comorbid depression in older diabetic Mexican Americans. Results from the Hispanic Established Population for the Epidemiologic Study of the Elderly survey. Diabetes Care. 1999;22(1):56–64.
49. Egede LE, Zheng D, Simpson K. Comorbid depression is associated with increased health care use and expenditures in individuals with diabetes. Diabetes Care. 2002;25(3):464–70.
50. Rubin RR, Peyrot M. Psychosocial problems in diabetes management: impediments to intensive self-care. Pract Diabetol. 1994;13:8–14.
51. Sclar DA, Robison LM, Skaer TL, Galin RS. Depression in diabetes mellitus: a national survey of office-based encounters, 1990–1995. Diabetes Educ. 1999;25(3):331–2, 335, 340.
52. Jacobson AM, Weinger K. Treating depression in diabetic patients: is there an alternative to medications? Ann Intern Med. 1998;129(8):656–7.
53. Kovacs M, Obrosky DS, Goldston D, Drash A. Major depressive disorder in youths with IDDM. A controlled prospective study of course and outcome. Diabetes Care. 1997;20(1):45–51.
54. Perez-Stable EJ, Miranda J, Munoz RF, Ying YW. Depression in medical outpatients. Underrecognition and misdiagnosis. Arch Intern Med. 1990;150(5):1083–8.
55. Rubin RR, Ciechanowski P, Egede LE, Lin EHB, Lustman PJ. Recognizing and treating depression in patients with diabetes. Curr Diab Rep. 2004;4:119–25.

56. Lustman PJ, Griffiths LS, Clouse RE. Recognizing and managing depression in patients with diabetes. In: Anderson BJ, Rubin RR, editors. Practical psychology for diabetes clinicians: how to deal with the key behavioral issues faced by patients and health care teams. Alexandria: American Diabetes Association; 1996. p. 143–54.
57. Gallo JJ, Rabins PV. Depression without sadness: alternative presentations of depression in late life. Am Fam Physician. 1999;60(3):820–6.
58. American Psychiatric Association. Diagnostic and statistical manual of mental disorders. 4th, text revision edn. Washington, DC: American Psychiatric Association; 2000.
59. Weinger K, Smaldone A. Psychosocial and educational implications of diabetic foot complications. In: Veves A, Giurini JM, LoGerfo FW, editors. The diabetic foot: medical and surgical management. 2nd ed. Totowa: Humana Press; 2006.
60. American Psychiatric Association. Diagnostic and statistical manual of mental disorders. 4th ed. Washington, DC: American Psychiatric Association; 1994.
61. Krishnan KR, Delong M, Kraemer H, Carney R, Spiegel D, Gordon C, et al. Comorbidity of depression with other medical diseases in the elderly. Biol Psychiatry. 2002;52(6):559–88.
62. Juurlink DN, Herrmann N, Szalai JP, Kopp A, Redelmeier DA. Medical illness and the risk of suicide in the elderly. Arch Intern Med. 2004;164(11):1179–84.
63. Suominen K, Henriksson M, Isometsa E, Conwell Y, Heila H, Lonnqvist J. Nursing home suicides-a psychological autopsy study. Int J Geriatr Psychiatry. 2003;18(12):1095–101.
64. Simon GE. Treating depression in patients with chronic disease: recognition and treatment are crucial; depression worsens the course of a chronic illness. West J Med. 2001; 175(5):292–3.
65. Thorpe L. Depression vs. dementia: how do we assess? The Canadian Review of Alzheimer's Disease and Other Dementias. 2009:17–21.
66. Sirey JA, Bruce ML, Alexopoulos GS, Perlick DA, Raue P, Friedman SJ, et al. Perceived stigma as a predictor of treatment discontinuation in young and older outpatients with depression. Am J Psychiatry. 2001;158(3):479–81.
67. Goldman LS, Nielsen NH, Champion HC. Awareness, diagnosis, and treatment of depression. J Gen Intern Med. 1999;14(9):569–80.
68. Glasser M, Gravdal JA. Assessment and treatment of geriatric depression in primary care settings. Arch Fam Med. 1997;6(5):433–8.
69. Corrigan PW, Swantek S, Watson AC, Kleinlein P. When do older adults seek primary care services for depression? J Nerv Ment Dis. 2003;191(9):619–22.
70. Peyrot M, Rubin RR, Siminerio LM. Physician and nurse use of psychosocial strategies in diabetes care: results of the cross-national Diabetes Attitudes, Wishes and Needs (DAWN) study. Diabetes Care. 2006;29(6):1256–62.
71. Beverly EA, Hultgren BA, Brooks KM, Ritholz MD, Abrahamson MJ, Weinger K. Understanding physicians' challenges when treating type 2 diabetic patients' social and emotional difficulties: a qualitative study. Diabetes Care. 2011;34(5):1086–8.
72. Schwenk TL. Diagnosis of late life depression: the view from primary care. Biol Psychiatry. 2002;52(3):157–63.
73. Gallo JJ, Anthony JC, Muthen BO. Age differences in the symptoms of depression: a latent trait analysis. J Gerontol. 1994;49(6):P251–64.
74. American Diabetes Association. Standards of medical care in diabetes – 2011. Diabetes Care. 2011;34 Suppl 1:S11–61.
75. Joiner Jr TE, Walker RL, Pettit JW, Perez M, Cukrowicz KC. Evidence-based assessment of depression in adults. Psychol Assess. 2005;17(3):267–77.
76. Yesavage JA, Brink TL, Rose TL, Lum O, Huang V, Adey M, et al. Development and validation of a geriatric depression screening scale: a preliminary report. J Psychiatr Res. 1982; 17(1):37–49.
77. Yesavage JA. Geriatric depression scale. Psychopharmacol Bull. 1988;24(4):709–11.
78. Onega LL. Content validation of the depressive symptom assessment for older adults. Issues Ment Health Nurs. 2008;29(8):873–94.
79. Navarro B, Andres F, Parraga I, Morena S, Latorre JM, Lopez-Torres J. Approach to major depression in old people. Int Psychogeriatr. 2010;22(5):733–8.

80. Lopez-Torres-Hidalgo JD, Galdon-Blesa MP, Fernandez-Olano C, Escobar-Rabadan F, Montoya-Fernandez J, Boix-Gras C, et al. Design and validation of a questionnaire for the detection of major depression in elderly patients. Gac Sanit. 2005;19(2):103–12.
81. Alexopoulos GS, Abrams RC, Young RC, Shamoian CA. Cornell scale for depression in dementia. Biol Psychiatry. 1988;23(3):271–84.
82. Alexopoulos GS, Abrams RC, Young RC, Shamoian CA. Use of the Cornell scale in nondemented patients. J Am Geriatr Soc. 1988;36(3):230–6.
83. Radloff LS. The CES-D scale: a self-report depression scale for research in the general population. Appl Psychol Meas. 1977;1(3):385–401.
84. Beck AT, Steer RA. Internal consistencies of the original and revised Beck Depression Inventory. J Clin Psychol. 1984;40(6):1365–7.
85. Rakovac I, Gfrerer RJ, Habacher W, Seereiner S, Beck P, Risse A, et al. Screening of depression in patients with diabetes mellitus. Diabetologia. 2004;47(8):1469–70.
86. Bech P. Quality of life in the psychiatric patient. London: Mosby-Wolfe; 1998.
87. Bech P. Male depression: stress and aggression as pathways to major depression. In: Dawson A, Tylee A, editors. Depression: social and economic timebomb. London: BMJ Books; 2001. p. 63–6.
88. Kroenke K, Spitzer RL, Williams JB. The PHQ-9: validity of a brief depression severity measure. J Gen Intern Med. 2001;16(9):606–13.
89. Kieffer KM, Reese RJ. A reliability generalization study of the Geriatric Depression Scale. Educ Psychol Meas. 2002;62:969–94.
90. Stiles PG, McGarrahan JF. The Geriatric Depression Scale: a comprehensive review. J Clin Geropsychol. 1998;4:89–110.
91. Burke WJ, Nitcher RL, Roccaforte WH, Wengel SP. A prospective evaluation of the Geriatric Depression Scale in an outpatient geriatric assessment center. J Am Geriatr Soc. 1992;40(12): 1227–30.
92. Peach J, Koob JJ, Mary JK. Psychometric evaluation of the Geriatric Depression Scale (GDS): supporting its use in health care settings. Clin Gerontol. 2001;23:57–68.
93. Lyness JM, Noel TK, Cox C, King DA, Conwell Y, Caine ED. Screening for depression in elderly primary care patients. A comparison of the Center for Epidemiologic Studies-Depression Scale and the Geriatric Depression Scale. Arch Intern Med. 1997;157(4): 449–54.
94. Gerety MB, Williams Jr JW, Mulrow CD, Cornell JE, Kadri AA, Rosenberg J, et al. Performance of case-finding tools for depression in the nursing home: influence of clinical and functional characteristics and selection of optimal threshold scores. J Am Geriatr Soc. 1994;42(10): 1103–9.
95. Sutcliffe C, Cordingley L, Burns A, Mozley CG, Bagley H, Huxley P, et al. A new version of the geriatric depression scale for nursing and residential home populations: the geriatric depression scale (residential) (GDS-12R). Int Psychogeriatr. 2000;12(2):173–81.
96. Shah A, Phongsathorn V, Bielawska C, Katona C. Screening for depression among geriatric inpatients with short versions of the Geriatric Depression Scale. Int J Geriatr Psychiatry. 1996;11:915–8.
97. Rinaldi P, Mecocci P, Benedetti C, Ercolani S, Bregnocchi M, Menculini G, et al. Validation of the five-item geriatric depression scale in elderly subjects in three different settings. J Am Geriatr Soc. 2003;51(5):694–8.
98. Gori C, Appolinio I, Riva P, Spiga D, Ferrari A, Trabucchi M. Using a single question to screen for depression in the nursing home. Arch Gerontol Geriatr. 1998;6(Suppl): 235–40.
99. Jongenelis K, Pot AM, Eisses AM, Gerritsen DL, Derksen M, Beekman AT, et al. Diagnostic accuracy of the original 30-item and shortened versions of the Geriatric Depression Scale in nursing home patients. Int J Geriatr Psychiatry. 2005;20(11):1067–74.
100. Ott BR, Fogel BS. Measurement of depression in dementia: self vs. clinician rating. Int J Geriatr Psychol. 1992;7:899–904.

101. Onalaja D, Sikaborfori T, Jainer AK. Differentiating depression from dementia in the elderly. Geriatr Med. 2004;34:67–71.
102. Bedard M, Molloy DW, Squire L, Minthorn-Biggs MB, Dubois S, Lever JA, et al. Validity of self-reports in dementia research: the Geriatric Depression Scale. Clin Gerontol. 2003; 26:155–63.
103. Burke WJ, Houston MJ, Boust SJ, Roccaforte WH. Use of the Geriatric Depression Scale in dementia of the Alzheimer type. J Am Geriatr Soc. 1989;37(9):856–60.
104. Heisel MJ, Duberstein PR. Suicide prevention in older adults. Clini Psychol Sci Pract. 2005; 12:242–59.
105. Sheikh JI, Yesavage JA, Brooks 3rd JO, Friedman L, Gratzinger P, Hill RD, et al. Proposed factor structure of the Geriatric Depression Scale. Int Psychogeriatr. 1991;3(1):23–8.
106. Hamilton M. A rating scale for depression. J Neurol Neurosurg Psychiatry. 1960;23:56–62.
107. Sunderland T, Alterman IS, Yount D, Hill JL, Tariot PN, Newhouse PA, et al. A new scale for the assessment of depressed mood in demented patients. Am J Psychiatry. 1988;145(8):955–9.
108. Ownby RL, Harwood DG, Acevedo A, Barker W, Duara R. Factor structure of the Cornell Scale for Depression in Dementia for Anglo and Hispanic patients with dementia. Am J Geriatr Psychiatry. 2001;9(3):217–24.
109. Burns A, Lawlor B, Craig S. Rating scales in old age psychiatry. Br J Psychiatry. 2002;180:161–7.
110. Kohout F. The pragmatics of survey field work among the elderly. In: Wallace R, Woolson R, editors. The epidemiological study of the elderly. New York: Oxford University Press; 1992. p. 99–119.
111. Kohout FJ, Berkman LF, Evans DA, Cornoni-Huntley J. Two shorter forms of the CES-D (Center for Epidemiological Studies Depression) depression symptoms index. J Aging Health. 1993;5(2):179–93.
112. Gellis ZD. Assessment of a brief CES-D measure for depression in homebound medically ill older adults. J Gerontol Soc Work. 2010;53(4):289–303.
113. Beck AT, Ward CH, Mendelson M, Mock J, Erbaugh J. An inventory for measuring depression. Arch Gen Psychiatry. 1961;4:561–71.
114. Beck AT, Steer RA, Ball R, Ranieri W. Comparison of Beck Depression Inventories -IA and -II in psychiatric outpatients. J Pers Assess. 1996;67(3):588–97.
115. Segal DL, Coolidge FL, Cahill BS, O'Riley AA. Psychometric properties of the Beck Depression Inventory II (BDI-II) among community-dwelling older adults. Behav Modif. 2008;32(1):3–20.
116. Jefferson AL, Power DV, Pope M. Beck Depression Inventory-II (BDI-II) and the Geriatric Depression Scale (GDS) in older women. Clin Gerontol. 2000;22:3–12.
117. Lustman PJ, Clouse RE, Griffith LS, Carney RM, Freedland KE. Screening for depression in diabetes using the Beck Depression Inventory. Psychosom Med. 1997;59(1):24–31.
118. Bech P, Olsen LR, Kjoller M, Rasmussen NK. Measuring well-being rather than the absence of distress symptoms: a comparison of the SF-36 Mental Health subscale and the WHO-Five Well-Being Scale. Int J Methods Psychiatr Res. 2003;12(2):85–91.
119. Awata S, Bech P, Koizumi Y, Seki T, Kuriyama S, Hozawa A, et al. Validity and utility of the Japanese version of the WHO-Five Well-Being Index in the context of detecting suicidal ideation in elderly community residents. Int Psychogeriatr. 2007;19(1):77–88.
120. Bonsignore M, Barkow K, Jessen F, Heun R. Validity of the five-item WHO Well-Being Index (WHO-5) in an elderly population. Eur Arch Psychiatry Clin Neurosci. 2001;251 Suppl 2:II27–31.
121. Allgaier AK, Liwowsky I, Kramer D, Mergl R, Fejtkova S, Hegerl U. Screening for depression in nursing homes: validity of the WHO (Five) Well-Being Index. Neuropsychiatr. 2011;25(4):208–15.
122. Awata S, Bech P, Yoshida S, Hirai M, Suzuki S, Yamashita M, et al. Reliability and validity of the Japanese version of the World Health Organization-Five Well-Being Index in the context of detecting depression in diabetic patients. Psychiatry Clin Neurosci. 2007;61(1):112–9.

123. Zimet GD, Dahlem NW, Zimet SG, Farley GK. The Multidimensional Scale of Perceived Social Support. J Pers Assess. 1988;52:30–41.
124. Zimet GD, Powell SS, Farley GK, Werkman S, Berkoff KA. Psychometric characteristics of the Multidimensional Scale of Perceived Social Support. J Pers Assess. 1990;55(3–4):610–7.
125. Phelan E, Williams B, Meeker K, Bonn K, Frederick J, Logerfo J, et al. A study of the diagnostic accuracy of the PHQ-9 in primary care elderly. BMC Fam Pract. 2010;11:63.
126. Lowe B, Unutzer J, Callahan CM, Perkins AJ, Kroenke K. Monitoring depression treatment outcomes with the Patient Health Questionnaire-9. Med Care. 2004;42(12):1194–201.
127. van Steenbergen-Weijenburg KM, de Vroege L, Ploeger RR, Brals JW, Vloedbeld MG, Veneman TF, et al. Validation of the PHQ-9 as a screening instrument for depression in diabetes patients in specialized outpatient clinics. BMC Health Serv Res. 2010;10:235.
128. Adler AI, Boyko EJ, Ahroni JH, Stensel V, Forsberg RC, Smith DG. Risk factors for diabetic peripheral sensory neuropathy. Results of the Seattle Prospective Diabetic Foot Study. Diabetes Care. 1997;20(7):1162–7.
129. Aiello LP, Gardner TW, King GL, Blankenship G, Cavallerano JD, Ferris 3rd FL, et al. Diabetic retinopathy. Diabetes Care. 1998;21(1):143–56.
130. Bethel MA, Sloan FA, Belsky D, Feinglos MN. Longitudinal incidence and prevalence of adverse outcomes of diabetes mellitus in elderly patients. Arch Intern Med. 2007;167(9):921–7.
131. Rein DB, Zhang P, Wirth KE, Lee PP, Hoerger TJ, McCall N, et al. The economic burden of major adult visual disorders in the United States. Arch Ophthalmol. 2006;124(12):1754–60.
132. Rizvi AA. Management of diabetes in older adults. Am J Med Sci. 2007;333(1):35–47.
133. Stratton IM, Adler AI, Neil HA, Matthews DR, Manley SE, Cull CA, et al. Association of glycaemia with macrovascular and microvascular complications of type 2 diabetes (UKPDS 35): prospective observational study. BMJ. 2000;321(7258):405–12.
134. Croxson SC, Price DE, Burden M, Jagger C, Burden AC. The mortality of elderly people with diabetes. Diabet Med. 1994;11(3):250–2.
135. Haffner SM, Lehto S, Ronnemaa T, Pyorala K, Laakso M. Mortality from coronary heart disease in subjects with type 2 diabetes and in nondiabetic subjects with and without prior myocardial infarction. N Engl J Med. 1998;339(4):229–34.
136. Kuusisto J, Mykkanen L, Pyorala K, Laakso M. NIDDM and its metabolic control predict coronary heart disease in elderly subjects. Diabetes. 1994;43(8):960–7.
137. Standl E, Balletshofer B, Dahl B, Weichenhain B, Stiegler H, Hormann A, et al. Predictors of 10-year macrovascular and overall mortality in patients with NIDDM: the Munich General Practitioner Project. Diabetologia. 1996;39(12):1540–5.
138. Wei M, Gaskill SP, Haffner SM, Stern MP. Effects of diabetes and level of glycemia on all-cause and cardiovascular mortality. The San Antonio Heart Study. Diabetes Care. 1998;21(7):1167–72.
139. Zigmond AS, Snaith RP. The hospital anxiety and depression scale. Acta Psychiatr Scand. 1983;67(6):361–70.
140. Derogatis LR. BSI 18: brief symptom inventory. Administration, scoring and procedures manual. Minneapolis: National Computer Systems, Inc; 2000.
141. Anderson RM, Fitzgerald JT, Funnell MM, Gruppen LD. The third version of the Diabetes Attitude Scale. Diabetes Care. 1998;21(9):1403–7.
142. Jacobson AM, the DCCT Research Group. The diabetes quality of life measure. In: Bradley C, editor. Handbook of psychology and diabetes. London: J. Wiley; 1994.
143. Jacobson AM, de Groot M, Samson JA. The evaluation of two measures of quality of life in patients with type I and type II diabetes. Diabetes Care. 1994;17(4):267–74.
144. Polonsky WH, Anderson BJ, Lohrer PA, Welch G, Jacobson AM, Aponte JE, et al. Assessment of diabetes-related distress. Diabetes Care. 1995;18(6):754–60.
145. Velligan D, Prihoda T, Dennehy E, Biggs M, Shores-Wilson K, Crismon ML, et al. Brief psychiatric rating scale expanded version: how do new items affect factor structure? Psychiatry Res. 2005;135(3):217–28.
146. Flemenbaum A, Zimmermann RL. Inter- and intra-rater reliability of the Brief Psychiatric Rating Scale. Psychol Rep. 1973;32(3):783–92.

147. Lachar D, Bailley SE, Rhoades HM, Espadas A, Aponte M, Cowan KA, et al. New subscales for an anchored version of the Brief Psychiatric Rating Scale: construction, reliability, and validity in acute psychiatric admissions. Psychol Assess. 2001;13(3):384–95.
148. Gary TL, Safford MM, Gerzoff RB, Ettner SL, Karter AJ, Beckles GL, et al. Perception of neighborhood problems, health behaviors, and diabetes outcomes among adults with diabetes in managed care: the Translating Research Into Action for Diabetes (TRIAD) study. Diabetes Care. 2008;31(2):273–8.
149. Whooley MA, Avins AL, Miranda J, Browner WS. Case-finding instruments for depression. Two questions are as good as many. J Gen Intern Med. 1997;12(7):439–45.
150. Durso SC. Using clinical guidelines designed for older adults with diabetes mellitus and complex health status. JAMA. 2006;295(16):1935–40.

Chapter 8
Screening for Depression in People with Diabetes in Primary Care

Margaret A. Stone and Paramjit S. Gill

Abstract This chapter considers the question of screening for depression in people with diabetes in primary care. Criteria for assessing the validity of screening are reviewed, together with national and international recommendations and selected research studies, with particular emphasis on relevance to primary care. A specific screening strategy currently being implemented in primary care in the UK is outlined. The need for rigorous evaluation of screening initiatives is highlighted, and a key conclusion is that case-finding alone is unlikely to be effective in terms of improving patient outcomes unless considered and applied in the context of overall case management.

Keywords Diabetes mellitus • Depression • Primary care • Screening • Criteria Guidelines • Outcomes

Introduction

The scale of the problem of undetected disease was highlighted many years ago, in a community setting, by the findings of the "Peckham Experiment" which began in London, UK, in the 1930s. In this study, conducted in the purpose-built Pioneer Health Centre, a defined population underwent annual medical checks and families

M.A. Stone, B.A. (Hons), Ph.D. (✉)
Department of Health Sciences, University of Leicester,
Leicester, UK
e-mail: mas20@le.ac.uk

P.S. Gill, DM, FRCGP, FHEA
Primary Care Clinical Sciences, University of Birmingham,
Birmingham, UK
e-mail: p.s.gill@bham.ac.uk

C.E. Lloyd et al. (eds.), *Screening for Depression and Other Psychological Problems in Diabetes*,
DOI 10.1007/978-0-85729-751-8_8, © Springer-Verlag London 2013

were observed. In 1970, a paper was published following earlier reports of the findings of the Peckham Experiment. This paper was pertinently titled "Periodic Overhaul of the Uncomplaining" [1]. The author, drawing from data for 1,000 families, noted that:

> ...of all those overhauled, only 10% were found to be without any clinically discoverable disorders. There were some 25–30% who knew they had some disease; less than half of these were under medical treatment at the time of examination. The remaining examinees (some 65–70%) all had some pathological disorder of which they were unaware, or which they ignored.

In 1963, Last introduced the notion of the "iceberg of disease," much of which lies submerged [2]. Identification of submerged, latent disease through screening or "case-finding" is an attractive concept but one with potential for inappropriate or ineffective application. In 1968, the World Health Organization (WHO) published Wilson and Junger's *Principles and Practice of Screening for Disease* [3]. In the preface to this document, the authors commented that in the developed world, where a higher level of resources is available compared to the developing countries:

> ...it would seem that the practice of screening for disease should be widespread. That it is not so to the extent that might be expected is due to a number of factors, among them the cost of screening and the tendency of the medical profession to wait for patients rather than actively to look for disease in the population. Another factor undoubtedly is inadequate knowledge of the principles and practice of screening for disease.

In their paper, Wilson and Junger [3] presented a list of ten "principles of early disease detection" which comprise global recommendations for assessing the validity of current or proposed screening strategies (Box 8.1). Although these criteria were formulated many years ago, they are still much cited and remain relevant and applicable to the question of the validity of screening (Box 8.1).

Box 8.1: Principles of Early Disease Detection: World Health Organization Criteria as First Described by Wilson and Junger [3]

1. The condition should be an important health problem.
2. There should be an accepted treatment for patients with recognized disease.
3. Facilities for diagnosis and treatment should be available.
4. There should be a recognizable latent or early symptomatic stage.
5. There should be a suitable test or examination.
6. The test should be acceptable to the population.
7. The natural history of the condition, including development from latent to declared disease, should be adequately understood.
8. There should be an agreed policy on whom to treat as patients.
9. The cost of case-finding (including diagnosis and treatment of patients diagnosed) should be economically balanced in relation to possible expenditure on medical care as a whole.
10. Case-finding should be a continuous process and not a "once and for all" project.

These ten principles underpin the more recent national guidelines produced by the National Screening Committee in the UK [4], which include some additional recommendations, for example, emphasizing the need to consider potential psychological harm:

> The benefit from the screening programme should outweigh the physical and psychological harm (caused by the test, diagnostic procedures and treatment).

The question of validity will be considered throughout this chapter, which describes and reflects on a specific screening strategy: identification of depression in people with diabetes through primary care providers. The chapter will focus mainly on this strategy as recommended and implemented in the UK, but some reference will also be made to other settings. Although type 1 and type 2 diabetes are distinct conditions, they will be considered together under the term "diabetes," except where specified, since much of the relevant literature and policy refers to the combined group of people with one of these two conditions.

Burden of Diabetes Management in Primary Care

People with type 2 comprise the majority of overall diabetes cases, and recent years have seen a shift in care of people with diabetes from hospital to primary care management [5]. This is a common trend throughout the developed world, although factors related to the overall organization of medical care in different countries are likely to have some influence on the way in which the management of people with diabetes is shared between primary and specialist care providers. In the UK, most people with type 2 diabetes are now managed in primary care at family practices, known as general practices in the UK. Management is provided by general practitioners (primary care doctors) and practice nurses. Findings from a study using data from 108 UK general practices from 1994 to 1996 indicated that two-thirds of people with type 2 diabetes were being managed in primary care alone [6], and this proportion is now likely to be even higher.

In general, in type 2 diabetes, only people with treatment-resistant poor glycemic control and those requiring insulin initiation (where expertise is not available at their general practice) are likely to be referred for management in secondary care in the UK. In some settings, referral to "intermediate care" providers (doctors and nurses with specialist training who see patients in a community setting) may also be available as an alternative to hospital management. Primary care health professionals may also be the sole care providers for people with type 1 diabetes, but there is a stronger likelihood of these patients being managed principally in secondary care. Even where people with diabetes are seen periodically by hospital specialists, their management is likely to be on a "shared care" basis, with general practices providing management support between hospital appointments. In the UK, most people with diabetes therefore attend their general practice for all or some part of their management.

Screening in a Primary Care Setting

Since most people with diabetes are seen in primary care for diabetes management (and also for other health issues), this setting could be considered highly appropriate for screening people with diabetes for unrecognized depression. This consideration could be said to support the validity of screening in primary care in respect of facilities for diagnosis (Box 8.1, Principle 3). In more general terms, the argument for screening for depression in people with diabetes is supported by the fact that evidence (including evidence from primary care research) suggests that there is a high level of latent disease (Box 8.1, Principle 4), since a high proportion of cases of depression in people with diabetes remain unrecognized. The authors of one review have suggested that depression is recognized and appropriately treated in fewer than 25% of depressed people with diabetes [7], while another study also found similarly low rates of recording of psychological problems in the medical notes of people identified as having anxiety, depression, and diabetes-related emotional problems [8]. Preliminary reporting of the findings of a screening study conducted in an ethnically diverse primary care setting in the UK also indicated higher rates of unrecognized major depression (Hospital Anxiety and Depression Scale scores of 11 or above) in people with diabetes compared to those without; undiagnosed depression was also noted to be more frequent in people of South Asian origin compared to white Europeans [9].

Importance of Depression in People with Diabetes Managed in Primary Care

Diabetes is a very common condition, and the increased prevalence of depression in people with diabetes is supported by two meta-analyses [10, 11], the more recent of which found that depression affects 10–20% of people with type 2 diabetes [11]. Overall, therefore, the combination of diabetes and depression can be said to occur with sufficient frequency for it to be considered an "important health problem" (Box 8.1, Principle 1) in respect of the number of people affected. It has been suggested, however, that depression may be more common in people with diabetes who are under the care of hospital physicians compared to those managed by primary care providers. A study conducted in three hospital diabetes outpatient clinics in the Netherlands, for example, identified high rates of depression in people with diabetes managed in these secondary care settings [12]. The authors found evidence of depressive affect, in 25% and 30% (men and women respectively) of participants with type 1 diabetes and in 35% and 38% (men and women respectively) of those with type 2 diabetes. In contrast, an earlier community-based study of people with type 2 diabetes, also conducted in the Netherlands, identified a lower (16.9%) overall prevalence of pervasive depression, with even lower rates (7.8%) in those with no chronic disease comorbidity [13]. Although most people with diabetes are managed in primary care, as described above, it could be argued that probable lower prevalence of depression in people who have not been referred to hospital specialists is a factor to be taken into account when considering the most appropriate setting for screening. This consideration may be relevant in terms of the seriousness of the problem, cost-effectiveness and, possibly, acceptability (Box 8.1, Principles 1, 9 and 6 respectively).

In terms of gravity, it is clear that depression per se has a serious impact on health outcomes including quality of life. In people with diabetes, there is some evidence of additional negative consequences including poorer glycemic control [14]. Although the relationship between diabetes and depression requires further clarification, particularly in terms of the probable two-way process of cause and effect, the nature and development of depression in general could be said to be "adequately understood" (Box 8.1, Principle 7). For people with diabetes who also have depression (recognized or unrecognized), the consequences of this comorbidity are potentially serious regardless of the primary or secondary care setting in which their diabetes is managed.

Managing Depression in People with Diabetes in Primary Care

There are accepted medical and psychological treatments for depression (Box 8.1, Principle 2). In the UK, guidance relevant to the question of "who to treat," for depression (Box 8.1, Principle 8) is available through the National Institute for Health and Clinical Excellence (NICE), which recommends a stepped-care approach [15] including recommendations relevant to people with different levels of depressive symptoms (Table 8.1).

The importance of monitoring and treating sub-threshold depressive symptoms has been highlighted by a study conducted in the Netherlands which found that, in patients with diabetes and sub-threshold depression, higher baseline anxiety and depression levels appeared to be associated with higher rates of developing major depression during 2 years of follow-up [16].

The stepped-care approach to the management of depression (Table 8.1) recommended in the UK provides a framework for managing those people who have been diagnosed with depression. This includes treatment options that, for most people, are provided in the same primary care setting as screening (Box 8.1, Principle 3). The Improving Access to Psychological Therapies (IAPT) program in the UK is designed to offer people (including, but not limited to, those with diabetes) access to psychological interventions such as cognitive behavioral therapy. Most primary care areas of England now have some level of access to services provided by this program [17]. Continuity of care is known to influence the acceptability of healthcare provision. If we extend the notion of acceptability of screening procedures (Box 8.1, Principle 6) to cover the combined processes of screening

Table 8.1 Management of diabetes: the stepped-care approach to depression management proposed by the UK National Institute for Health and Clinical Excellence

Step	Target cases	Intervention
1	All known and suspected presentations of depression	Assessment, support, psycho-education, active monitoring and referral for further assessment and interventions
2	Persistent sub-threshold depressive symptoms; mild to moderate depression	Low-intensity psychosocial interventions, psychological interventions, medication, and referral for further assessment and interventions
3	Persistent sub-threshold depressive symptoms or mild to moderate depression with inadequate response to initial interventions; moderate and severe depression	Medication, high-intensity psychosocial interventions, combined treatments, collaborative care, and referral for further assessment and interventions
4	Severe and complex depression; risk to life; severe self-neglect	Medication, high-intensity psychological interventions, electroconvulsive therapy, crisis service, combined treatments, multi-professional and inpatient care

Adapted from: NICE clinical guideline 90 – depression [15]

and treatment-if-diagnosed, continuity resulting from both processes being conducted in a familiar primary care setting may have a positive influence on the extent to which these processes are perceived as acceptable.

Recommendations for Identifying Depression in People with Diabetes

There are validated methods of assessing depression status (Box 8.1, Principle 5), for example, using self-report questionnaires or diagnostic interviews. These methods are suitable for use in a range of settings, including primary care. Recognizing that identification of depressive symptoms in people with diabetes is an important consideration, many diabetes management guidelines produced in different countries now include a recommendation highlighting the need to be alert to the possibility of undiagnosed depression and its consequences. These guidelines do not necessarily include recommendations regarding formal screening strategies. The guideline for management of type 1 diabetes, produced by NICE in the UK [18], for example, recommends that:

> Members of the professional teams providing care or advice to adults with diabetes should be alert to the development or presence of clinical or sub-clinical depression and/or anxiety, in particular where someone reports or appears to be having difficulties with self-management.

The UK national guideline for management of type 2 diabetes [19] states the following and also refers the reader to the NICE guideline for the management of depression [15]:

> People with Type 2 diabetes with psychological and/or depressive disorders should be identified by continuing professional awareness, and managed in accordance with current national guidelines.

Relevant guidance is provided in a position statement from the American Diabetes Association (ADA), which is frequently used as a reference point throughout the world. This statement [20] includes the following recommendations regarding psychosocial assessment in the management of people with diabetes, although it should be noted that the evidence levels cited are relatively low (C: Supportive evidence from poorly controlled or uncontrolled studies or E: Expert consensus or clinical experience):

- Assessment of psychological and social situation should be included as an on-going part of the medical management of diabetes. (E)
- Psychosocial screening and follow-up should include, but is not limited to, attitudes about the illness, expectations for medical management and outcomes, affect/mood, general and diabetes-related quality of life, resources (financial, social and emotional), and psychiatric history. (E)
- Screen for psychosocial problems such as depression and diabetes-related distress, anxiety, eating disorders, and cognitive impairment when self-management is poor. (C)

The ADA recommendations also suggest that:

> Key opportunities for screening of psychosocial status occur at diagnosis, during regularly scheduled management visits, during hospitalization, at discovery of complications, or when problems with glucose control, quality of life, or adherence are identified.

In addition, they propose that:

> It is preferable to incorporate psychological assessment and treatment into routine care rather than waiting for identification of a specific problem or deterioration in psychological status.

The approach recommended is based on incorporating psychological assessment into routine management of diabetes and is essentially opportunistic rather than formally pro-active. It is implied that the setting for this type of opportunistic screening would most commonly be where the patient is primarily managed either in the community or in specialist care, but that it could also occur in other settings, for example, during an inpatient hospital stay. Additional guidance provided by the ADA includes suggesting that there are a range of "issues which are known to have an impact on self-management and health outcomes." Those mentioned include attitudes to the illness, expectations relating to management, and affect/mood. The guideline document also highlights the fact that there are a number of relevant screening tools available.

Guidelines produced by the International Diabetes Federation (IDF) for global use in the management of type 2 diabetes [21] include recommendations relating to three levels of diabetes care: minimal, standard and comprehensive. Guidance for standard care includes recommendations that healthcare providers should:

> Explore the social situation, attitudes, beliefs and worries related to diabetes and self-care issues.
> Assess well-being and psychological status (including cognitive dysfunction) periodically, by questioning or validated measures (e.g. WHO-5)
> Discuss the outcomes and clinical implications with the person with diabetes, and communicate findings to the other team members where appropriate.

For minimal care, it is recommended that care providers should:

> Be alert to signs of cognitive, emotional behavioural and social problems which may be complicating self-care, particularly where diabetes outcomes are sub-optimal.

Recommendations for comprehensive care suggest that, in addition to periodic assessment and discussion as for standard care, healthcare providers could:

> ...use additional measures ... and computer-based automated scoring systems. The mental health specialist in the team would be able to provide a more comprehensive (neuro) psychological assessment, if indicated.

The WHO-5 questionnaire referred to in the IDF recommendations for standard care cited above is a five-question instrument provided by the WHO. The use of the terms "periodically" and "questioning or validated measures" in the IDF recommendations are imprecise and, therefore, open to interpretation. This could be taken to suggest a flexible rather than a formal "screening program" approach to identification of depressive symptoms in people with diabetes. Alternatively, the general recommendations provided in the IDF guideline, and in the other guidelines cited above, could be interpreted as offering a framework for the design of a more formal screening program involving specified frequency and standardized methods of assessment and follow-up.

Effectiveness and Feasibility of Screening: Current Evidence

In this section, illustrative (rather than exhaustive) evidence relevant to the topic of the effectiveness and feasibility of screening for depression in people with diabetes will be considered, with particular emphasis on the relevance of this evidence to screening in primary care settings. There is some evidence to support the theoretical appropriateness of screening for depression in people with diabetes, for example, on the basis of that this is an "important problem" as outlined above. However, if the available treatments are likely to be ineffective in populations targeted for screening, the implementation of screening lacks justification. A number of studies have confirmed that treatment of depression, once diagnosed, can be effective in people with diabetes. These studies have included both pharmacologic and non-pharmacologic interventions. To cite two examples, a study involving the use of fluoxetine in people with type 1 or type 2 diabetes demonstrated improvements related to depression [22], and a combination of cognitive behavior therapy and supportive diabetes education led to benefits both in terms of depression and glycemic control in people with type 2 diabetes recruited from primary care [23]. However, transferability of results from research to real world settings is always a factor to be taken into account in considering the clinical implications of trial findings. In addition, in both these studies, assessment of depression using questionnaires and diagnostic interviewing was used to determine eligibility for the study and to measure outcomes, rather than for screening. In their paper which includes an overview of evidence relating to the effectiveness of treatment for depression in people with diabetes, one of Rubin et al.'s [7] conclusions is that:

> Controlled trials suggest antidepressant medication or psychotherapy can relieve depression in people with diabetes, and that effective treatment may also contribute to improved glycaemic control.

In spite of some theoretical support for the notion of screening for depression in people with diabetes, it needs to be demonstrated that this strategy is both feasible and effective when implemented. To be confirmed as appropriate, screening needs, for example, to be shown to be acceptable (Box 8.1, Principle 6); the screening test should be found to be effective in terms of case-finding in the target population and thus truly "suitable" (Box 8.1, Principle 5); and cost-effectiveness needs to be considered (Box 8.1, Principle 9).

There is currently a paucity of specific evidence within the literature regarding the acceptability and effectiveness of screening for depression in people with diabetes. Nevertheless, some evidence related to screening for depression in more general populations or people with other conditions (rather than specifically in people with diabetes) may be considered to be relevant. In a review collating evidence on this more general topic [24], the authors presented findings derived from a Cochrane systematic review of randomized controlled trials that included the use of instruments for case-finding or screening for depression in non-mental health settings. The authors specifically sought to determine the effectiveness of using such instruments without additional enhancement of care; they considered the impact of screening or case-finding on recognition, management and outcomes of depression. Meta-analysis indicated that pro-active case-finding had a significant but modest impact on recognition of depression (relative risk 1.27). At more detailed level, they noted that depression-specific scales appeared to be more effective than more general instruments and that preselection of higher-risk patients increased the effect size. The impact of screening in terms of increasing the use of any intervention for depression (relative risk 1.30) narrowly failed to reach significance, and the effect of screening on prescription of antidepressants (relative risk 1.20) was non-significant. Additionally, findings from a small number of studies suggested no overall impact of screening on depression outcomes (nonsignificant standardized mean difference –0.02). In summarizing their findings, the authors concluded that they:

> … found no substantial effect of screening or case-finding instruments on the overall recognition rates of depression, the management of depression by clinicians or on depression outcomes.

They noted that these findings were true for both primary care and hospital settings and suggested that their study emphasizes that screening without additional enhancements to the overall organization of care is not justified, concluding that:

> … screening without other systematic changes to improve depression management is unlikely to improve outcomes.

A recent multicenter randomized controlled trial can be considered particularly relevant, as it specifically involved people with diabetes [25]. This study also found that depression screening, using questionnaires with feedback to physicians, had a limited impact on depression-related healthcare utilization or outcomes (depression and diabetes-related distress) compared to usual care. In a qualitative study, a series of interviews was conducted with people with depression identified by a primary care screening program [26]. Although this study was not specific to people with diabetes, it is pertinent to note that a high proportion of those interviewed were reluctant to accept their diagnosis of depression. The authors suggest that patients' views about depression should be explored prior to offering diagnosis and treatment. The findings from these two studies support the need to consider screening in the context of the overall organization of care, including access to psychological counseling.

Questions addressed by the authors of a review relating to depression screening in people with cardiovascular disease [27] included the accuracy of screening tools; these authors identified 11 relevant studies and found a wide range in terms of both sensitivity (the ability to accurately identify cases with depression) and specificity (the ability to accurately identify cases without depression). Sensitivity ranged from 39% to 100% (median 84%) and specificity from 58% to 94% (median 79%). Although the authors described these levels as reasonable, they also noted that there were few examples of screening tools or screening tool thresholds with demonstrated accuracy in more than one sample of patients. In addition, they noted that none of the studies had considered possible harm caused by screening, for example, the impact of false-positive results (including adverse effects and cost implications), the cost and inconvenience of additional assessments, and inappropriate labeling. The authors of this review found evidence of modest improvements in symptoms of depression, but no improvements in cardiovascular outcomes, as a result of treatment for depression. They were unable to identify any studies providing evidence specifically about the impact of depression screening on outcomes (for depression or cardiovascular disease) in people with cardiovascular disease. Overall, therefore, they were unable to provide any evidence of a specific link between screening for depression and improved outcomes, in the category of patients reviewed.

In a study conducted in 38 general practices in three areas of the UK, Kendrick et al. [28] used anonymized medical records data to consider the relationship between patients' scores on depression questionnaires (BDI-II or HADS) and rates of antidepressant drug prescribing and referrals to specialist care providers. In this study, the two questionnaires were used to assess severity of symptoms in patients who had already received a new diagnosis of depression, rather than as screening tools for case-finding. In addition, the cases included were not limited to people with diabetes. Nevertheless, the findings of this study are of some relevance in that they suggested that the two questionnaires performed inconsistently and also in terms of highlighting the role of clinical judgment in general practitioners' decisions about drug treatment or referral for depression. In their discussion, the authors suggest that these decisions are unlikely to be based on questionnaire scores alone and that:

> The question then is which is more accurate in terms of predicting the need for treatment, general practitioners' clinical judgement or questionnaire measures?

They also suggest that future research might usefully include asking practitioners to rate their certainty of diagnosis and the need for treatment prior to administration of questionnaires.

Although there is a lack of evidence regarding the impact of screening for depression (as a distinct intervention) on outcomes in people with diabetes, some studies provide a degree of relevant insight because they have included screening as part of a broader, multifaceted intervention for people with diabetes. In a randomized controlled trial conducted in the Netherlands [29], the authors investigated the impact of a complex intervention involving monitoring of depression status and follow-up. A diabetes specialist nurse assessed psychological well-being in intervention group participants using a computerized questionnaire, and the score was used to facilitate a follow-up discussion. The nurses carrying out the intervention had been trained by psychologists to discuss the result with the patient in an exploratory, nonjudgmental manner. Findings from this study indicated some modest favorable effects of the intervention on psychological well-being (mood) but no impact on glycemic control. The study was conducted in a hospital outpatient setting, which limits its relevance to the main focus of this chapter, since people with diabetes managed in secondary care are likely to have more intensive treatment, more complications and/or poorer glycemic control compared to people treated solely in primary care. More importantly, in considering the relevance of this study to the specific topic under consideration, where an intervention has more than one component, the contribution of specific components (such as the screening or monitoring initiative regardless of follow-up) is likely to be unclear.

The Pathways study [30] was conducted in primary care patients with diabetes in the USA. The two-stage depression screening process was used to assess eligibility for the randomized trial rather than as part of the intervention being investigated. The two strategies used for identifying trial participants were: initial screening using a mailed invitation to complete the Patient Health Questionnaire-9 (PHQ-9) followed by a longer symptom checklist (SCL-90) administered 2 weeks later by telephone to those with PHQ-9 scores of 10 or more. A total of 4,839 initial questionnaires were returned and 1,038 (21%) were eligible for the second stage screening, based on PHQ-9 scores. Of the 851 people who were screened using the SCL-90, 375 (8% of those who returned initial questionnaires) met the criteria for recruitment to the trial (SCL-90 score of >1.1) and 329 agreed to participate. The collaborative care intervention involved initial patient choice regarding two treatment options (medication or problem solving treatment) and a stepped-care approach. Over a 12-month period, people in the intervention group showed significantly greater improvements in terms of depressive symptoms, but no improvements in glycemic control.

In a narrative review article, Pouwer considered the question: *should we screen for emotional distress in type 2 diabetes*? [31]. The scope of the review was not limited to depression but also included anxiety and diabetes-specific emotional problems such as worries about future complications, concerns about food, feelings of guilt and shame, non-acceptance of the diagnosis, and distressing social interactions. The findings of the review article are, nevertheless, salient to the question of screening for depression in people with diabetes. The author of this review highlights the problem of under-detection and subsequent under-treatment of depression, anxiety and diabetes-specific distress and suggests that the use of screening tools can help to increase detection rates but that more research is needed "to determine which tools should be used for this purpose, by whom and how often." Consistent with the conclusions from other studies mentioned above, the author also suggests that:

> …the most important message of this Review is that case-finding alone does not improve diabetes outcomes. Crucially, screening efforts should be embedded in collaborative care approaches…

Overall, findings derived from reviews and individual studies suggest that more research-based evidence is needed to support the case for the widespread introduction of screening for depression in people with diabetes in primary care, or indeed in other settings. A recurrent message is that screening alone is unlikely to have a strong impact on patient outcomes unless case-finding is linked to other aspects of patient management.

Screening for Depression in People with Diabetes in UK Primary Care

In this section, one model of screening for depression in people with diabetes in primary care will be described and considered in more detail. This model is the one currently recommended and implemented in primary care in the UK. The underlying motivation for encouraging pro-active screening or case-finding for depression in diabetes is based on potential health and well-being benefits to patients and possible cost savings at system level (Box 8.1, Principle 9) linked to improved outcomes, for

Table 8.2 Quality and Outcomes Framework indicators: depression in people with diabetes and/or coronary heart disease

Indicator		Standard (basis of eligibility for points) (%)	Maximum points
DEP 1	The percentage of patients on the diabetes register and/or the CHD register for whom case finding for depression has been undertaken on one occasion during the previous 15 months using two standard screening questions	40–90	8
DEP 2	In those patients with a new diagnosis of depression, recorded between the preceding 1 April to 31 March, the percentage of patients who have had an assessment of severity at the outset of treatment using an assessment tool validated for use in primary care	40–90	25
DEP 3	In those patients with a new diagnosis of depression and assessment of severity recorded between the preceding 1 April to 31 March, the percentage of patients who have had a further assessment of severity 5–12 weeks (inclusive) after the initial recording of the assessment of severity. Both assessments should be completed using an assessment tool validated for use in primary care	40–90	20

example, reduced levels of diabetes-related complications. However, when considering a specific case-finding strategy, it is necessary to consider not only the limited evidence base for this rationale (see above) but also potential advantages and limitations of the specific model in question.

The Quality and Outcomes Framework (QOF) is a voluntary incentive scheme which operates in the UK, whereby general practices providing primary care receive payments based on the extent to which specified targets are met [32, 33]. The QOF measures of achievement are based on evidence from research, and they cover four domains: clinical (indicators related to specific health conditions); organizational (e.g. process indicators regarding record keeping and patient information); patient experience (e.g. related to length of consultation); and additional services (such as child health surveillance). Payments are made retrospectively for points achieved during the previous year; the average predicted payment per general practice for 2011/2012 in England has been estimated as £130.51 per point achieved [34]. The QOF indicators relevant to identifying and classifying depression in people with diabetes are shown in Table 8.2. It should be noted that the first of these indicators (DEP1) relates to people with coronary heart disease as well as those with diabetes, and the other two (DEP2, DEP3) refer to all patients with a new diagnosis of depression, including (but not restricted to) those with diabetes.

Screening for depression in line with the recommendations suggested by the QOF indicators is not a formal policy and is probably most appropriately described as an ad hoc strategy. The QOF indicators do not prescribe a specific method of ensuring that all people with diabetes are regularly assessed for possible depression. It is not suggested that there should be a national or local system for inviting patients to attend specifically for a "depression screening" appointment, for example, in the way that women in the UK are called in to their general practice specifically for a smear test for cervical cancer screening. It is unlikely that this type of approach would be adopted for depression screening in people with diabetes, who are generally reviewed regularly by their healthcare providers for overall management of their chronic condition. A screening approach involving a dedicated appointment would be time consuming for busy primary healthcare providers working within a system where limited time is available to care for the overall patient population. Moreover, in general terms, screening has potential for causing anxiety in those invited, and it could be surmised that a strategy involving a dedicated appointment would also be less acceptable to patients, who might assume that their mental stability was being questioned if invited to attend their general practice specifically for assessment of depressive symptoms. Incorporating this assessment into a routine chronic disease review is likely to be less challenging for patients and therefore more acceptable (Box 8.1, Principle 6).

Primary care providers in the UK use computerized record-keeping systems to record information about their patients, including demography, current and past medical history, consultations, test results, prescribed medications and referrals. These computer systems generally offer an "alert" facility to remind general practitioners and practice nurses to carry out certain tasks, for example, rechecking smoking status or carrying out a blood pressure check. This option offers a very practical means of ensuring that patients with diabetes have an annual assessment of possible depressive symptoms, thus facilitating the implementation of a case-finding strategy that is a continuous process rather than a "once and for all" project (Box 8.1, Principle 10).

The two questions referred to in QOF indicator DEP 1 (Table 8.2) are known as the Patient Health Questionnaire-2 (PHQ-2) and are worded as follows:

- During the last month, have you often been bothered by feeling down, depressed or hopeless?
- During the last month, have you often been bothered by having little interest or pleasure in doing things?

In a study involving a range of patients, rather than specifically those with diabetes, attending15 general practices in New Zealand, these two questions had a sensitivity of 97% and specificity of 67% for identifying depression [35]. There are three assessment tools "validated for use in primary care" (QOF indicators DEP2 and DEP3): the Patient Health Questionnaire-9 (PHQ-9); the Beck Depression Inventory, second edition (BDI-II); and the Hospital Anxiety and Depression Scale (HADS). These questionnaires are all designed to identify depression in three categories: mild, moderate, and severe and are described in more detail elsewhere in this book. Most general practices in the UK have opted to use the PHQ-9, which has nine questions

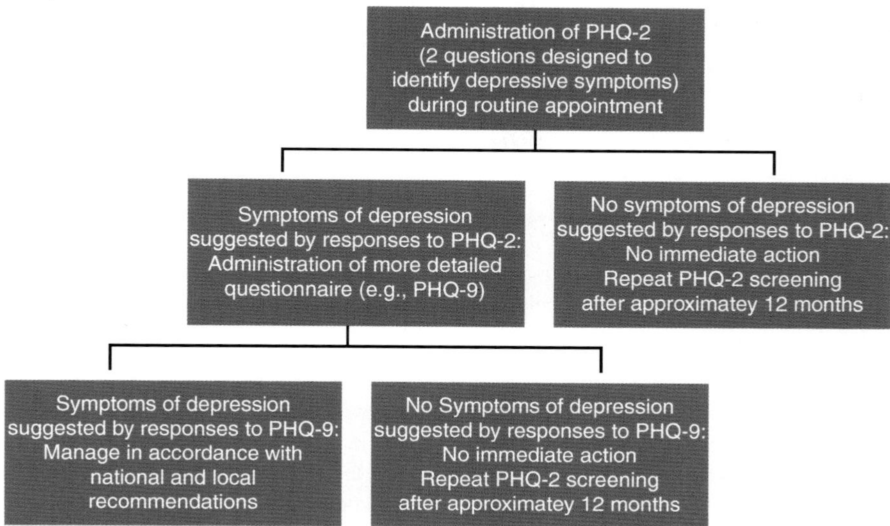

Fig. 8.1 Screening for depression in UK primary care

about frequency relating to a series of indicators of possible depression. There is also a tenth question about how difficult any of these problems have made daily activities. Selecting the PHQ-9 rather than the BDI-II or HADS is likely to be largely pragmatic since it is relatively short and there is no license fee payable for obtaining or administering this questionnaire (Fig. 8.1).

Time constraints are an important factor to take into account when considering the utility of the current UK strategy for screening people with diabetes for depression. Healthcare providers must be assumed to have the overall best interests of their patients in mind when carrying out their daily tasks, but they face pressures related to busy workloads in an increasingly demanding health service. These pressures may potentially have an impact on the quality of the process of screening, both at the initial stage using the PHQ-2 and for follow-up assessment using the longer PHQ-9. Criteria for assessing the validity of screening proposed by the UK National Screening Committee [4] specifically raise the issue of quality control, specifying that:

> There should be a plan for managing and monitoring the screening programme and an agreed set of quality assurance standards.

The QOF incentive scheme provides a method of measuring the extent to which criteria are met in numerical terms. These data are freely available both at national, local (primary care trust), and general practice level [36]. Results for 2009/2010 (Table 8.3) indicate high levels of achievement in terms of meeting the standards set for the three QOF indicators related to identification and management of depression. These findings are encouraging in relation to efforts to improve levels of recognition and severity monitoring of depression in primary care.

Table 8.3 Average achievement rates in England for QOF depression indicators for the year 2009/2010 (based on data for 8,305 general practices)

Indicator	Summary description[a]	Underlying achievement[b] (%)
DEP1	Initial screening using two questions (PHQ-2)	88.3
DEP2	Follow-up screening using more detailed questionnaire	91.8
DEP3	Reassessment	70.1

Source of data: [36]
[a]See Table 8.2 for full description of indicator
[b]Percentage of eligible patients in whom criterion was met

Although compliance with the QOF recommendations is monitored in this way, the quality of the process is assumed rather than specifically considered. Indeed, quality control is more generally a potential issue in relation to healthcare process measures, where there is scope for variations in the administration of that process. More objective measurements relating to outcomes such as glycated hemoglobin levels are less susceptible to variation relating to the quality of the measurement. Unless additional time to carry out the process of screening is scheduled within a regular diabetes review appointment, there is a danger that this activity, though recorded as completed, may have been carried out rapidly and, therefore, less effectively. Moreover, the fact that the screening processes in question are linked to an incentive scheme may increase the danger of these processes becoming a "box-ticking" exercise where time constraints exert an influence. Scheduling additional, dedicated time into the appointment has implications related to costs, which may not be covered by the modest payments received through the QOF incentive scheme. Even if money is available, securing additional staff capacity may be problematic. Furthermore, cost implications need to be considered in the overall context of finite resources for healthcare provision (Box 8.1, Principle 9).

Linking case-finding to an incentive scheme raises the issue of possible manipulation of data. There is some evidence salient to this consideration, although this relates to the overall implementation of the QOF scheme rather than specifically to depression screening in diabetes. This evidence suggests that the fact that the UK depression screening strategy is linked to incentives is likely to have very limited impact in terms of compromising the validity of this strategy. Doran et al. have presented their analysis of data relating to "exception reporting" whereby a range of criteria is used to exclude certain patients from those included in QOF reporting [37]. These authors considered the possibility that primary care providers might use the practice of "gaming" to inappropriately exclude patients for whom QOF targets have not been met but found little evidence that this occurs frequently. In a qualitative study, doctors and nurses working in UK general practices were interviewed to explore their perceptions about the effects of the introduction of the QOF incentive scheme. A few interviewees admitted to occasional data manipulation, but most suggested that they endeavored to apply the incentive scheme framework honestly and ethically [38].

A further potential limitation of the UK screening approach based on self-report questionnaires concerns the appropriateness of the questionnaires for use in different populations, including people from different educational and ethnic backgrounds. The PHQ-9, for example, was developed in English speaking individuals and has not been validated in other cultural groups. If the PHQ-2 questions or the full PHQ-9 questionnaire are administered through an interpreter (who may be the healthcare provider, another member of the general practice staff or someone, such as a family member, accompanying the patient), there is potential for inconsistency and reduced validity.

An additional factor which has potential for influencing the quality of the process of carrying out depression screening UK primary care in accordance with the policy suggested by the QOF targets relates to the perceptions of the person carrying out the screening. The extent to which this person believes in the validity of the questionnaires for identifying depression may have an influence, as may their views regarding the added value of this type of screening over normal clinical management, including their knowledge of individual patients (involving factors such as personal and social circumstances and overall medical history). It is possible that the type of screening process recommended could be seen as a challenge to the value of healthcare providers' general clinical skills. In the interview study cited above [38], some respondents described their perceptions that other aspects of patient care could be compromised by pressure to concentrate on those areas covered by the incentive scheme, and some doctors were unhappy with the impact of standardization and "box-ticking" on their "caring role."

Although developments in terms of screening for depression in people with diabetes in the UK have shown some promise (Table 8.3), many questions remain unanswered regarding the validity of the ad hoc strategy being implemented in line with QOF recommendations. While this case-finding process in the UK does not constitute a formal screening program, factors such as implications for patients and health-related resource usage (particularly healthcare professional time) mean that criteria for assessing the validity of screening are, nevertheless, relevant. It may be particularly pertinent to note that one of the criteria for validity of screening proposed by the UK National Screening Committee [4] states that:

> Clinical management of the condition and patient outcomes should be optimised in all health care providers prior to participation in a screening programme.

It could be argued that the introduction of the current screening strategy in primary care prior to full implementation of the IAPT program [17] in all areas constitutes failure to comply with this criterion. At this early stage, evidence is lacking regarding the effectiveness of the current UK screening strategy in terms of outcomes, including outcomes specific to people with diabetes. Rigorous evaluation is needed and this should incorporate qualitative explorations of acceptability, including the implications of "labeling," and quantitative evaluations relating to short- and long-term health outcomes, absolute costs, and cost-effectiveness.

Conclusions

Overall, additional evidence-based clarification is required to support the case for widespread screening for depression in people with diabetes in primary care settings. While the importance of this combination of conditions is well established, it remains to be shown that formal pro-active screening has benefits over improved methods of incorporating recognition and management of depression into routine models of care of people with diabetes. Optimal strategies for screening or case-finding require further investigation, but it is important to acknowledge that the impact of any such strategies on patient outcomes is likely to be minimal unless combined with effective overall case management, including the availability of appropriate services and expertise. In primary care this may include availability within this setting and, also (additionally or alternatively), effective referral opportunities.

References

1. Pearse IH. Periodic overhaul of the uncomplaining. J R Coll Gen Pract. 1970;20:146–52.
2. Last JM. The iceberg "completing the clinical picture" in general practice. Lancet. 1963;ii:28–31.
3. Wilson JMG, Junger G. Principles and practice of screening for disease. Public Health Papers, 34. Geneva: World Health Organisation; 1968.
4. National Screening Committee. The UK National Screening Committee's criteria for appraising the validity, effectiveness and appropriateness of a screening programme. London: HMSO; 2003.
5. Goyder EC, McNally PG, Drucquer M, Spiers N, Botha JL. Shifting of care for diabetes from secondary to primary care, 1990–1995: review of general practices. BMJ. 1998;316:1505–6.
6. Khunti K, Ganguli S. Who looks after people with diabetes: primary or secondary care? J R Soc Med. 2000;93:183–6.
7. Rubin RR, Ciechanowski P, Egede LE, Lin EHB, Lustman PJ. Recognizing and treating depression in patients with diabetes. Curr Diab Rep. 2004;4:119–25.
8. Pouwer F, Beekman ATF, Lubach C, Snoek FJ. Nurses' recognition and registration of depression, anxiety and diabetes-specific emotional problems in outpatients with diabetes mellitus. Patient Educ Couns. 2006;60:235–40.
9. Ali S, Taub NA, Stone MA, Davies MJ, Skinner TC, Khunti K. Ethnic differences in the prevalence and recognition of depression in a primary care population with and without type 2 diabetes. Diabetologia. 2010;53 Suppl 1:S21.
10. Anderson RJ, Freedland KE, Clouse RE, Lustman PJ. The prevalence of co-morbid depression in adults with diabetes. Diabetes Care. 2001;24:1069–78.
11. Ali S, Stone MA, Peters JL, Davies MJ, Khunti K. The prevalence of co-morbid depression in adults with type 2 diabetes: a systematic review and meta-analysis. Diabet Med. 2006;23:1165–73.
12. Pouwer F, Geelhoed-Duijvestijn PHLM, Tack CJ, Bazelmans E, Beekman A-J, Heine RJ, et al. Prevalence of depression is high in out-patients with type 1 or type 2 diabetes mellitus. Results from three out-patient clinics in the Netherlands. Diabet Med. 2010;27:217–24.
13. Pouwer F, Beekman ATF, Nijpels G, Dekker JM, Snoek FJ, Kostense PJ, et al. Rates and risks for co-morbid depression in patients with type 2 diabetes mellitus: results from a community-based study. Diabetologia. 2003;46:1124–6.

14. Lustman PJ, Anderson RJ, Freedland KE, De Groot M, Carney R, Clouse RE. Depression and poor glycaemic control: a meta-analytic review of the literature. Diabetes Care. 2000;23:934–42.
15. National Institute for Health and Clinical Excellence. Clinical guideline 90. Depression. The treatment and management of depression in adults. London: National Institute for Health and Clinical Excellence; 2009.
16. Bot M, Pouwer F, Ormel J, Slaets JP, de Jonge P. Predictors of incident major depression in diabetic outpatients with subthreshold depression. Diabet Med. 2010;27:1295–301.
17. Improving Access to Psychological Therapies (IAPT). Information available at: http://www.iapt.nhs.uk/about-iapt/. Last accessed Jan 2012.
18. National Institute for Clinical Excellence. Type 1 diabetes: diagnosis and management of type 1 diabetes in children, young people and adults. London: National Institute for Clinical Excellence; 2004.
19. National Collaborating Centre for Chronic Conditions. Type 2 diabetes: national clinical guideline for management in primary and secondary care (update). London: Royal College of Physicians; 2008.
20. American Diabetes Association. Standards of medical care in diabetes – 2011. Diabetes Care. 2011;34(1):S11–61.
21. International Diabetes Federation Clinical Guideline Task Force. Global guideline for type 2 diabetes. Brussels: International Diabetes Federation; 2005.
22. Lustman PJ, Freeland KE, Griffith LS, Clouse RE. Fluoxetine for depression in diabetes. A randomised double-blind placebo-controlled trial. Diabetes Care. 2000;23:618–23.
23. Lustman PJ, Griffith LS, Freedland KE, Kissel SS, Clouse RE. Cognitive behaviour therapy for depression in type 2. Diabetes mellitus a randomized, controlled trial. Ann Intern Med. 1998;129:613–21.
24. Gilbody S, Sheldon T, House A. Screening and case-finding instruments for depression: a meta-analysis. CMAJ. 2008;178:997–1003.
25. Pouwer F, Tack CJ, Geelhoed-Duijvestijn PH, Bazelmans E, Beekman AT, Heine RJ, et al. Limited effect of screening for depression with written feedback in outpatients with diabetes mellitus: a randomised controlled trial. Diabetologia. 2011;54:741–8.
26. Wittkampf KA, van Zwieten M, Smits FTh, Schene AH, Huyser J, van Weert HC. Patients' view on screening for depression in general practice. Fam Pract. 2008;25:438–44.
27. Thombs BD, de Jonge P, Coyne JC, Whooley MA, Frasure-Smith N, Mitchell AJ, et al. Depression screening and patient outcomes in cardiovascular care. A systematic review. JAMA. 2008;300: 2161–71.
28. Kendrick T, Dowrick C, McBride A, Howe A, Clarke P, Maisey S, et al. Management of depression in UK general practice in relation to scores on depression severity questionnaires: analysis of medical record data. BMJ. 2009;338:b750.
29. Pouwer F, Snoek FJ, van der Ploeg HM, Adèr HJ, Heine RJ. Monitoring of psychological well-being in outpatients with diabetes. Effects on mood, HbA1c, and the patient's evaluation of diabetes care: a randomized controlled trial. Diabetes Care. 2001;24:1929–35.
30. Katon WJ, Von Korff M, Lin EHB, Simon G, Ludman E, Russo J, et al. The pathways study. A randomized trial of collaborative care in patients with diabetes and depression. Arch Gen Psychiatry. 2004;61:1042–9.
31. Pouwer F. Should we screen for emotional distress in type 2 diabetes mellitus? Nat Rev Endocrinol. 2009;5:665–71.
32. Doran T, Fullwood C, Gravelle H. Pay for performance programs in family practices in the United Kingdom. N Engl J Med. 2006;335:375–84.
33. National Institute for Health and Clinical Excellence. Information available at: http://www.nice.org.uk/aboutnice/qof/qof.jsp. Last accessed Jan 2012.
34. British Medical Association. Information available at: http://www.bma.org.uk/images/focusqofpaymentsoct2011/_v4_tcm41–209913.pdf. Last accessed Jan 2012.
35. Arroll B, Khin N, Kerse N. Screening for depression in primary care with two verbally asked questions: cross sectional study. BMJ. 2003;327:1144–6.

36. Information Commissioners. Information available from: http://signposting.ic.nhs.uk/?k=QOF/. Last accessed Jan 2012.
37. Doran T, Fullwood C, Reeves D, Gravelle H, Roland M. Exclusion of patients from pay-for-performance targets by English physicians. N Engl J Med. 2008;359:274–84.
38. Maisey S, Steel N, Marsh R, Gillam S, Fleetcroft R, Howe A. Effects of payment for performance in primary care: qualitative interview study. J Health Serv Res Policy. 2008;13:133–9.

Chapter 9
Screening in Secondary Care

Mirjana Pibernik-Okanović and Dea Ajduković

Abstract Secondary care institutions provide advanced treatment of diabetic patients whose health is threatened by a chronic course of diabetes or severe comorbidities. Elevated depressive symptoms and emotional distress are common in persons facing the advanced stages of diabetes, including its late complications. Depressive affect increases the risk for developing complications and vice versa, as suffering from complications increases the risk for elevated depressive symptoms. Therefore, secondary diabetes services specialized for treating microvascular and macrovascular complications have a particular responsibility to detect patients' emotional problems early and to properly address them. Integrating screening for emotional problems with appropriate treatment options is crucial for improving outcomes. A stepped care approach may meet individual patients' needs and be feasible in a busy clinical practice.

Keywords Screening in secondary care reening • Depression • Diabetes-related distress • Secondary care • Diabetes complications • Treatment for depression Stepped care •

Introduction

Specialized diabetes clinics organized at a secondary health care level either as outpatient clinics or as hospital departments deal with patients who have more complex health problems than primary care patients. These problems may reflect a more

M. Pibernik-Okanović, Ph.D. (✉) • D. Ajduković, M.Sc.
Deporment of Clinic for Diabetic Complications, Vuk Vrhovac University Clinic for Diabetes, Merkur Teaching Hospital, Zagreb, Croatia
e-mail: pibernik@idb.hr; dea.ajdukovic@idb.hr

C.E. Lloyd et al. (eds.), *Screening for Depression and Other Psychological Problems in Diabetes*,
DOI 10.1007/978-0-85729-751-8_9,

chronic course of diabetes, including life-threatening complications, somatic comorbidities, and psychological risk factors, such as poor self-care or a presence of psychological symptoms. In order to achieve the purpose of secondary and tertiary prevention, defined as improving patients' quality of life by reducing the severity and progression of diabetes, it is necessary to recognize and manage the associated psychological risk factors. Recent reports indicate that patients whose psychological needs are adequately addressed are more satisfied with their care and overall functioning [1, 2]. Early detection and treatment of diabetes complications is considered crucial for slowing the progressive course of this chronic illness, thus protecting patients' functional capacity and their emotional well-being. During the last several decades, a large body of research has accumulated, providing evidence that the course and the prognosis of diabetes are not associated only with biomedical determinants but also with psychosocial factors. Consequently, a biopsychosocial model of care has been increasingly advocated to effectively treat diabetes and to properly meet patients' needs.

People with diabetes who have developed complications, and especially those with multiple complications, have been shown to be at an increased risk of psychological problems – most frequently depression and diabetes-related emotional distress. Therefore, special importance should be given to screening for emotional difficulties when treating individuals suffering from diabetic retinopathy, neuropathy, nephropathy, erectile dysfunction, diabetic foot, cardiovascular disease, or a combination of several of these complications. Since these patients are likely to be referred to secondary health care services specialized for treating microvascular and macrovascular abnormalities, recognizing and properly addressing emotional problems should be considered inherent to the diagnostic and treatment process at this level of health care.

This chapter aims to summarize data on the interaction between diabetes complications and psychological problems and to suggest practical approaches that might improve both patients' physical and psychological outcomes.

Why Is Screening for Depressive Symptoms Important in Patients with Complications?

A Bidirectional Relationship of Depression and Diabetes Complications

The increased prevalence of depressive symptoms in patients with diabetes compared to individuals without diabetes [3] has been found to be consistently associated with diabetes complications including retinopathy, neuropathy, nephropathy, macrovascular complications, and erectile dysfunction [4]. Both cross-sectional and prospective studies have confirmed the adverse interaction between depression and diabetes outcomes [5, 6]. In one study which took place over a 5-year period, patients with major depression were compared with nondepressed diabetic patients and had a 36% higher risk for developing advanced microvascular complications such as end-stage renal disease and blindness and a 25% higher risk for developing advanced macrovascular complications such as cardiac infarction or stroke, even after adjusting for baseline diabetes severity and self-care activities [7]. The severity of depression has also been associated with an increased risk of incident retinopathy, as well as with time to incident retinopathy, suggesting that improving depression treatment in patients with diabetes could contribute to the prevention of diabetic retinopathy [8]. The risk of incident foot ulcers has been found to be increased twofold in individuals with comorbid depression compared to diabetic patients who are not depressed [9]. Depressed patients with diabetic neuropathy are more prone to developing first foot ulcers than nondepressed individuals, independently of biological risk factors and foot care [10]. Patients with diabetes and depression, compared to those with diabetes alone, have been found to have a greater risk for dementia, with one study showing a doubled incidence rate per 1,000 person-years during a 5-year follow-up [11]. Patients with major depression are also more frequently admitted to intensive care units and are hospitalized for longer periods [12] indicating that this comorbidity complicates the course of diabetes.

There is also strong evidence of an inverse association between diabetes complications and depression. Patients burdened by diabetes complications are more likely to develop depression than are those without complications, especially in the case of nephropathy and neuropathy [13]. Neuropathy-related symptoms, impairment in daily activities, and neuropathy-related changes in important roles are predictive of increases in depressive symptoms over time [14]. Depression is common in patients with erectile dysfunction, which reflects a continuous interplay between diabetes-related and psychological factors. Although severe erectile dysfunction is mainly related to the severity of diabetes, mild to moderate dysfunction has been found to be independent of clinical variables and associated with the severity of depressive symptoms only [15].

Current evidence on the interaction between diabetes complications and emotional problems suggests a bidirectional relationship, implying that emotional problems increase the risks for developing complications and that the presence of complications increases the risk for emotional problems (Fig. 9.1) [16, 17].

A series of biological, psychological, and behavioral factors might explain this interaction. Biological factors that could mediate the link between depression and poor vascular outcomes include HPA axis activity (increased cortisol secretion), the sympathetic nervous system (increased catecholamine release), proinflammatory and procoagulation responses (increased levels of cytokines or platelet/endothelial cell adhesion molecule-1), and heart rate variability. However, further research is needed to fully understand the interaction.

Psychosocial factors mediating the relationship between diabetes complications and depression encompass the emotional burden associated with facing the advanced stages of the illness, including functional impairment, pain, and adverse social implications. At least some of these factors are modifiable through medical and

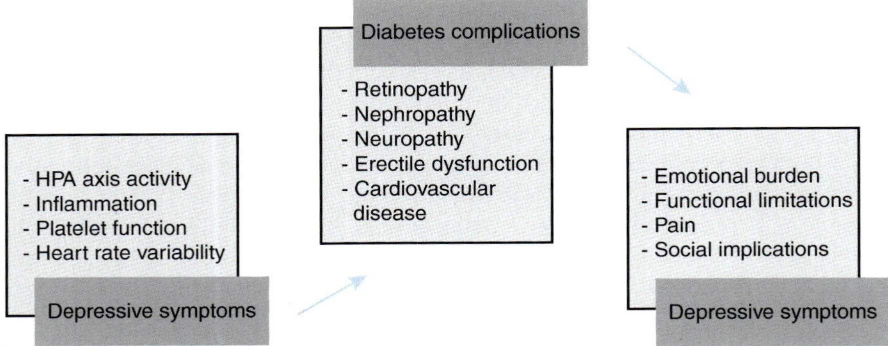

Fig. 9.1 The relation between depressive symptoms and hypothetical mechanisms that mediate them

psychosocial interventions, such as using medical support and psychological techniques to relieve pain. In light of that, regular screening for depressive symptoms is important in enabling timely and adequate interventions for depression, thus improving not only depression-related but also diabetes-related outcomes.

Why Is Screening for Depressive Symptoms Not Enough?

The Relevance of Diabetes-Related Emotional Distress

Patients reporting depressive symptoms frequently report emotional problems related to diabetes as well [18–21]. Moreover, recent research findings suggest that diabetes-related distress or significant emotional reactions to burdensome aspects of diabetes, such as threat of complications, are more common than depressive difficulties and more closely related to diabetes self-care and glycemic control [22, 23].

Diabetes-related distress has been shown to persist over time, especially in younger diabetic individuals, women, and those with complications and/or comorbidities [20]. Both objective indicators of disease severity and subjective ratings of impairment contribute to emotional distress in the affected individuals and, consequently, in developing more severe psychological symptoms. Also, perceived changes in disease intrusiveness over time may increase emotional distress, thus making the depressive symptoms in the affected individuals more severe [24].

Diabetes-related emotional problems and diabetes self-management are interrelated – high levels of emotional distress are associated with poor self-management of diabetes and vice versa; low self-efficacy in managing diabetes increases the emotional distress caused by it [25]. Since self-management of diabetes is one of the best predictors of diabetes outcomes, recognizing and properly addressing emotional

Table 9.1 Steps in recognizing psychological symptoms in patients treated at secondary care level

Who to screen?	Patients with painful neuropathy
	Patients with visual impairment
	Patients with erectile dysfunction
	Patients with renal failure
	Patients with diabetic foot and amputations
	Patients with a history of depression
When to screen?	At first clinical visit
	Every 6 months if screening results are positive
	After completing the recommended treatment
	Once a year if screening results are negative
What to screen for?	Depressive symptoms
	Emotional distress caused by diabetes
What instruments to use?	PHQ-2, CES-D, WHO-5
	PAID, PAID-5 (diabetes distress)

distress in patients who are at risk for complications, or have already developed them, is crucial for preventing adverse health outcomes and slowing their progression.

How to Implement Screening Procedures into the Clinical Care of Persons with Diabetic Complications?

Screening for depressive symptoms and diabetes-related emotional distress is a necessary first step in raising awareness of these frequent problems in patients treated at the secondary care level. Ideally, all diabetic patients should be screened for depression and diabetes-related emotional distress at their first clinical visit as part of a clinical assessment. However, in the often more realistic circumstances of limited resources and high patient load, efforts should be directed at the groups of patients who are most likely to need support, using the most efficient screening instruments available, at realistically set time intervals (Table 9.1).

Complications such as painful neuropathy, visual impairment, renal failure, diabetic foot and amputations, or erectile dysfunction are especially likely to impair the patients' functional ability, well-being, and mental health. Screening for these patients' depressive symptoms and emotional distress should be made a priority. The other group of patients who are likely to need additional support are those with a history of psychological and psychiatric difficulties. Given the high recurrence rate of depression, especially in diabetic patients, a history of depressive difficulties should be considered a strong indication that periodic screening for depression and diabetes distress is necessary.

After the initial screening, these patients should be screened annually at their regular diabetes checkups if their diabetes distress and depressive symptoms are not elevated, and at least every 6 months if they report elevated symptoms of diabetes distress and/or depression. If patients are included in a treatment program aimed at improving their psychological well-being, they should be rescreened after treatment and then at regular 12-month intervals.

However, screening itself is not likely to improve depression scores and has a limited impact on mental health utilization in patients with diabetes [26]. To improve its clinical utility, screening should be accompanied by:

(a) Inquiring into patients' needs for treatment
(b) Synchronizing screening with treatment recommendations
(c) Using a stepped care approach to ensure continuous follow-up

Inquiring into Patients' Needs for Receiving Professional Help in Mood-Related Difficulties

Not all patients facing emotional difficulties, either disease related or those that are a part of their broader life context, are willing to be comprehensively treated for their mental health problems. In our ongoing large study, 77% of female and 76% of male type 2 diabetes patients who screened positive for depression expressed a need for professional support with their symptoms [27]. This implies that approximately one-fourth to one-fifth of patients may prefer approaches which are not specific for depression but are rather incorporated into their usual diabetes treatment [28]. By using a screening instrument for depression which inquires not only into depressive symptoms but also into individual needs for treatment [29], the specificity of screening and its clinical utility have been shown to be improved. From a clinical point of view, knowing about patients' readiness to engage in treatment for emotional problems may help to individualize treatment and make it feasible from the patients' perspective. The modified Patient Health Questionnaire-Depression (PHQ-2) is given in Box 9.1.

Box 9.1: The Adjusted PHQ-2 Screening Instrument

1. During the past month have you often been bothered by feeling down, depressed, or hopeless?

   YES NO

2. During the past month have you often been bothered by having little interest or pleasure in doing things ?

   YES NO

2. Answer if you have responded "yes" to 1 or 2: is this something with which you would like help?

   YES NO

Combining Depression Screening with Interventions Proven to Be Effective and Feasible in Everyday Clinical Practice

According to the criteria for appraising the viability, effectiveness, and appropriateness of a screening program [30], an effective intervention should be available for the condition that is being sought. In the field of diabetes care, many psychological and pharmacological treatments, as well as collaborative care for depression, including options for both psychotherapy and pharmacotherapy, have been shown to be effective in treating patients with diabetes and depression. A meta-analysis by van der Feltz-Cornelis and colleagues [31] found 14 randomized controlled trials (RCT) with a total of 1,724 patients which dealt with the impacts of psychotherapeutic and pharmacological treatments on depression and diabetes-related outcomes. Depression treatment was shown to have a moderate effect on depression-related outcomes in people suffering from diabetes. In general, the effects of depression treatment were smaller on glycemic control than on mental health outcomes. Psychotherapeutic interventions demonstrated larger effects in improving glycemic control than did pharmacological interventions. However, the sizes of the particular studies were too small to generalize from these results. The authors concluded that the treatment of depression in people with diabetes is a necessary step to improve depressive symptoms, but in order to improve the general medical condition, including glycemic control, simultaneous attention to both conditions may be desirable.

This can be supported by the results of a recent study by Katon and colleagues [32]. Patients with poorly controlled diabetes, coronary heart disease, or both, and a coexisting depression were randomly assigned to either a usual-care group or an intervention group in which a medically supervised nurse, working with each patient's physician, provided guideline-based collaborative care management. Patients in the intervention group as compared to the controls had a greater 12-month improvement in HbA1c, LDL cholesterol, systolic blood pressure, and depression scores. They were also more likely to adjust insulin, antihypertensive, and antidepressant medication. Indicators of quality of life and treatment satisfaction were also higher in patients assigned to the intervention group. The study results suggest that an intervention involving collaborative and proactive follow-up which integrates the management of the medical and the psychological illness improved medical and depression outcomes in patients with multiple somatic conditions.

A recent systematic review of treatments for depression in patients with diabetes [33] confirmed that cognitive-behavioral therapy, antidepressant medications, and collaborative care are all effective in the treatment of depression in diabetes, but the efficacy of these treatments in improving glycemic control remains unclear. Taking into consideration the strong evidence of the association between depression and diabetes complications [4], and depression and diabetes self-management which is a very strong predictor of diabetes complications [34], the authors suggested novel treatment approaches that would integrate self-management training with strategies to decrease depressive symptoms. Such treatments may lead to a greater improvement in diabetes-related outcomes than depression treatment alone.

For example, in a trial of cognitive-behavioral therapy adapted to address diabetes-relevant behavior change [35], changes in both glycemic control and diabetes-related distress were achieved in poorly controlled type 1 patients as compared to control patients. These benefits were maintained over the 1 year of follow-up. Similar benefits were observed in a peer-delivered self-management intervention in type 2 diabetic patients; both diabetes-related distress and glycemic control improved relative to control subjects, and these improvements were maintained over 18 months [36].

The potential benefits of psychological interventions in patients with advanced diabetic complications were demonstrated in a study by Devins and colleagues [37]. A predialysis psychoeducational intervention was carried out in 297 patients with progressive renal disease who were expected to require renal replacement therapy within 6–18 months. The intervention arm of this prospective randomized trial included an interactive psychoeducational intervention, a printed booklet, and supportive telephone calls every 3 months. Time to dialysis therapy was significantly longer in the treated group as compared to individuals in usual diabetes care. The authors hypothesized that the underlying mechanisms involve the acquisition and implementation of illness-related knowledge.

Screening for both depression and diabetes-related distress and distinguishing between the two conditions has been increasingly advocated in the recent literature [38]. Also, besides identifying diabetes distress or depressive symptoms, clarifying the context in which patients' psychological problems have been generated is necessary for planning and adjusting interventions.

Embedding Depression Screening into a Stepped Care Approach Which Takes into Consideration Patients' Preferences for Different Treatment Modes

The decision as to which treatment is adjusted to particular individuals depends on their specific health condition (which complications they are coping with and how much objective impairment is involved, how they subjectively perceive their physical and psychological impairment) and their preferences regarding treatment. We can assume that some individuals would prefer receiving nonspecific support from their health care practitioners, while some would be motivated to engage into more comprehensive treatments. A step-by-step approach starting with treatments that are acceptable for the majority of patients who report depressive symptoms and proceeding with more complex ones in the case of nonresponsiveness (or severe initial difficulties) seems to be preferable. It can be considered justified not only from the perspective of patient-centered care but also from the cost-effectiveness perspective.

What Are the Steps in Responding to the Needs of Patients with Depression and/or Diabetes Distress?

When screening for depressive symptoms and diabetes distress, there are four possible combinations of results (Fig. 9.2):

- Negative for depression and diabetes distress
- Positive for depression, negative for diabetes distress
- Negative for depression, positive for diabetes distress
- Positive for both depression and diabetes distress

If the results for both depression and diabetes distress are negative, no further interventions are needed, aside from a regular reassessment on a yearly basis. If the screening instruments, however, indicate either depressive difficulties or diabetes-related distress, or both, action should be taken to ameliorate the patient's condition. These actions should be directed toward offering alternative treatment options that

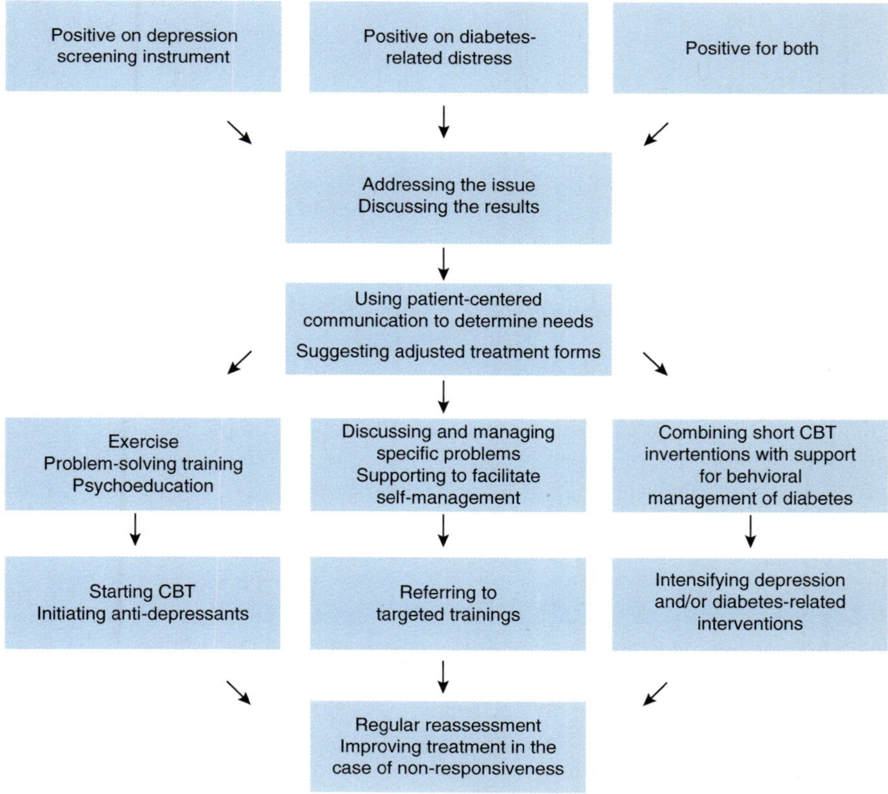

Fig. 9.2 Integrating screening with treatment options adjusted to patients' problems and needs

would better address the patient's difficulties and needs, either in managing mood, self-management of diabetes and its complications, or both. Communication in all steps of care should be patient centered. This entails acknowledging both the patient and the practitioner as individual persons through whose joint efforts and shared responsibility health benefits can be achieved [39].

As a first step, the issue of depression and diabetes distress should be addressed with the patient. He or she should be informed of their results on the screening instruments, which should be discussed in a patient-centered way. The difficulties and needs of the patient should be clarified in this discussion, including the patient's perceived need and motivation for further treatment. Even a brief discussion of the patient's subjective difficulties integrated into regular diabetes care can prove reassuring and motivating, as it acknowledges the patient's experience and emotions [38]. If the patient is interested in receiving further help, support and treatment options should be explained, and a recommendation of the type of treatment made based on the extent of their difficulties.

Elevated Depressed Mood on Screening

There are a number of interventions of varying intensity that can be utilized in providing help to patients who reported mood difficulties in screening instruments. The decision as to which interventions to offer should be made taking into consideration the patient's subjective need for help, his or her preference of the type of treatment, and the feasibility of the interventions in clinical practice. However, as serious psychopathology may underlie elevated depressive symptoms on screening instruments, an additional assessment of the intensity of the symptoms should be made. Validated and broadly used instruments such as CES-D or structured psychiatric interviews can be useful to achieve this [40].

Patients who suffer from mild depressive difficulties may benefit from less intensive forms of support. One option is exercise, a form of treatment that is increasingly gaining empirical support in the treatment of mild depression [41, 42]. Patients who prefer psychological approaches or who are unable to participate in exercise for various reasons (physical limitations or medical conditions) can be offered structured forms of psychological support such as psychoeducation or problem-solving training. The aim of such programs is to provide patients with the skills and support for self-help in depression. The leader of the group takes the role of a teacher, and not a psychotherapist, which means that health workers who are not primarily mental health professionals may successfully implement these interventions [43]. Both exercise and psychological support are typically offered as structured programs delivered in a group setting to maximize efficiency and foster social support. However, if there are specific patient needs and constraints or organizational constraints, they can be successfully carried out on an individual basis as well.

Patients who do not benefit from less intensive forms of support or whose initial difficulties warrant more intensive treatment may benefit from validated psychotherapeutic approaches, such as cognitive-behavioral therapy [44]. This type of treatment is typically provided by a formally trained professional in a group or individual setting and usually lasts for 12–16 one-hour sessions. If talking therapy on its own proves ineffective, antidepressant treatment should be introduced, either as the sole mode of treatment or, preferably, together with cognitive-behavioral therapy.

Elevated Diabetes Distress in Screening

In patients who screen positive for diabetes distress and not depressive symptoms, efforts should be directed toward improving diabetes-related issues while providing general psychosocial support. These patients' mood should be reassessed periodically.

The first step in reducing diabetes distress is to discuss issues that patients face in the course of their diabetes self-management. Such a discussion alone may foster self-management by keeping the patients motivated and by providing a feeling of support [37]. Simple treatment changes or providing information may prove useful in lessening the impact of the disease in the patients' everyday life. The distress of a patient who is concerned about his or her morning hyperglycemia may thus decrease with an adjustment in insulin regime; a patient who is worried about the effects of taking a lot of medication may be relieved by appropriate education about drug safety. These interventions may be successfully combined with diabetes reeducation geared toward improving and supporting self-management. Diabetes self-management education is successful both in achieving diabetes-related clinical improvements and in fostering psychological well-being [45] and quality of life [46]. Research has indicated [47] that many different formats of diabetes self-management education (in terms of group vs. individual format, number of contacts, who delivered the intervention, overall duration of the intervention, focus on knowledge vs. lifestyle) can be equally successful in achieving clinical results, provided that adequate time is spent with patients and that patients are actively engaged in the process.

Patients whose diabetes-related distress is associated with specific, well-defined factors should be offered targeted trainings and programs to help with these issues. Such patients may benefit from structured blood glucose awareness training [48] or stress management training [49].

The Combination of Elevated Depressive Symptoms with Elevated Diabetes-Related Distress in Screening

In patients who screen positive for both depressive symptoms and diabetes-related distress, treatment recommendations should start with short cognitive-behavioral therapy (CBT)-based interventions equally incorporating both depression-related and diabetes-related contents. A regular reassessment, optimally at a 6-month basis, is recommended in order to provide a proper follow-up of these vulnerable individuals. More intensive forms of treatment including CBT and/or antidepressants will be needed in case of persistent symptoms of depression or prolonged diabetes distress. Clinical attention should be directed toward understanding the interplay between depression and diabetes distress at an individual level, and tailored interventions should be provided if a patient does not respond to more general ones.

What if Comprehensive Interventions Are Not Feasible in Everyday Practice?

Comprehensive screening for psychological symptoms and agreeing about appropriate treatment modes in those who are found positive for depressive symptoms, diabetes-related distress, or both, might be difficult for health care practitioners in terms of time constraints and other treatment priorities. However, research data indicate that even a short inquiry into patients' mood state and their need to receive support may be helpful in recognizing depressive symptoms and identifying necessary steps to be taken. In a study by Ayalon and colleagues for example [50], elderly patients with diabetes were asked the single-item question: "Do you think you suffer from depression?" The results indicated that this had as good or even better sensitivity than other screens (83%) and could, accordingly, be used in detecting depression in older patients. When promoting simple emotion-focused interventions to support a patient's self-management of diabetes, Peyrot and Rubin [51] have suggested an easy, time-limited inquiry into depressive symptoms ("In the past 2 weeks have you felt depressed or lost interest or pleasure in things?") and when deciding whether the patient needs to be referred for treatment ("Would you like to talk with someone who could help you to resolve these problems?"). Such a step-by-step approach to psychosocial issues may facilitate patient-provider communication, thus improving outcomes.

In order to illustrate the dynamic relationship between psychological symptoms and diabetes-related issues, two case studies are given in Boxes 9.2 and 9.3.

Conclusion

There is convincing evidence that depressive symptoms and diabetic complications are interrelated, thus making screening for psychological symptoms in patients at risk for adverse health outcomes justified and needed. Although further research is necessary to clearly define how depression screening might be optimally incorporated into everyday clinical practice in order to improve both depression- and diabetes-related outcomes, there are undoubted clinical benefits of recognizing and properly addressing psychological problems. Patients treated at secondary care level are recommended to be screened and treated for depressive symptoms and diabetes-related distress as proposed in Fig. 9.2. This procedure includes screening for

Box 9.2: Case Report 1

The patient is a 48-year-old man who was diagnosed with type 1 diabetes when he was 20 years old. He was referred to a diabetes day hospital in a specialist diabetes clinic due to poor glycemic regulation (HbA1c=8.0%), neuropathy and retinopathy, and his unawareness of hypoglycemia. At the beginning of treatment, he was screened for depressive symptoms and diabetes distress, which were both significantly elevated (CES-D score=23, PAID score: emotional=75, food=60, treatment=75, social=0). He participated in a 5-day program of diabetes education that included psychoeducation. He was seen by a neurologist, and a diagnosis of diabetic vegetative neuropathy was made. For this reason, he was coached in raising his blood glucose awareness, and plans were made for introducing an insulin pump. At the end of his stay at the diabetes day hospital, his diabetes distress and depressive symptoms were significantly lower (CES-D score=16) but still called for attention. His GP was informed of the need for depression evaluation and treatment. In the process of introducing the insulin pump, the patient was repeatedly seen by a diabetologist and rescreened for depression and diabetes distress, his scores being negative on the screening instruments. He reported that he had started antidepressant medication prescribed by his GP and that he was feeling better. He was also very satisfied with insulin pump treatment, and his blood glucose regulation improved (HbA1c=6.4%). However, at a diabetologist checkup 18 months after his stay at the diabetes day hospital, his score on the depression screening instrument indicated severe depressive symptoms (CES-D=33), and his blood glucose levels were significantly higher (HbA1c=8.3%). He was interviewed by a clinical psychologist, to whom he reported that he felt profoundly depressed and had suicidal thoughts and plans. This prompted an evaluation by a liaison psychiatrist, who made a diagnosis of a recurrent depressive disorder. The patient was prescribed a new combination of antidepressant medication and was scheduled for frequent psychiatric reevaluations.

Box 9.3: Case Report 2

A 60-year-old man with a 21-year history of type 2 diabetes treated by a combination of insulin and oral hypoglycemic agents was routinely screened for depression by the PHQ-2 sent by mail. The returned reply indicated positive symptoms, and the patient expressed a need for receiving professional help. His health status at the time of depression screening was characterized by poor glycemic control (HbA1c=8.30%). Although he had been diagnosed with nonproliferative retinopathy 3 years before, he did not attend the recommended patient visits. The patient was married and worked as an administrator. He described his marital situation as supportive and his professional circumstances as stressful and burdensome.

In order to determine the severity of depression, a structured clinical interview based on the DSM-IV was administered by phone. There were no indicators of a clinical diagnosis of depression. The patient's score on the CES-D was 14, and the PAID score did not indicate emotional problems related to diabetes (sum score = 24). Since his mood was evaluated as subclinical depression, the patient was included in a 6-week psychoeducational course aimed at acquiring skills for self-managing depression. He attended the course regularly and afterward reported satisfaction with what he had learned. The course moderator's observations indicated that the patient was receptive to support coming from other group members but was not ready to practice using the CBT principles taught in the course. He did not complete his home exercises regularly and was prone to evaluating them as not being useful. The CES-D score after the course was unchanged [14]. Follow-up of depressive symptoms and glycemic control was agreed upon, and a 6-month follow-up visit was scheduled.

Three months after the end of the treatment, the patient asked for an individual consultation with a psychologist, explaining that his mood state was significantly worsened. He was faced with worries and obligations related to his mother's health problems which caused in him feelings of enormous helplessness and insecurity. He reported trying techniques he had learned during the course – recognizing negative thoughts, reframing, and relaxation techniques – but did not find them helpful. After two supportive appointments with the psychologist, one of which was carried out as a session with the patient and his wife together, the symptoms did not improve. An appointment with a psychiatrist was scheduled and pharmacotherapy was introduced. The patient now requires both a psychological and a diabetes follow-up. Prompts to self-monitor blood glucose and support for regular ophthalmological care have been provided.

depressive symptoms and diabetes-related distress, discussing the results with the patients, suggesting adjusted treatment forms, and regularly reassessing the symptoms. If comprehensive procedures like these are not feasible in busy clinical practice, even basic inquiry into patients' mood state and their need to be supported is considered promising in meeting individual needs and improving diabetes outcomes.

Important Points

- Psychological problems adversely affect the course of diabetes and its prognosis.
- Depressive symptoms and diabetes-related distress are common in patients suffering from diabetes complications.

- Patients with diabetes complications are likely to be referred to secondary health care services. Therefore, recognizing and properly addressing psychological problems should be inherent to diagnostic processes at this health care level.
- Screening itself is not likely to improve psychological and disease-related outcomes. Integrating it with patients' treatment-related needs and preferences is necessary to improve prognosis.
- Stepped care ranging from support to improving diabetes self-management to psychoeducation, cognitive-behavioral therapy, and pharmacological treatment can be recommended in meeting individual patients' needs

References

1. Katon WJ, Von Korff M, Lin EH, Simon G, Ludman E, Russo J, et al. The pathways study: a randomized trial of collaborative care in patients with diabetes and depression. Arch Gen Psychiatry. 2004;61(10):1042–9.
2. Williams Jr JW, Katon W, Lin EH, Noel PH, Worchel J, Cornell J, et al. The effectiveness of depression care management on diabetes-related outcomes in older patients. Ann Intern Med. 2004;140(12):1015–24.
3. Anderson RJ, Freedland KE, Clouse RE, Lustman PJ. The prevalence of comorbid depression in adults with diabetes: a meta-analysis. Diabetes Care. 2001;24(6):1069–78.
4. de Groot M, Anderson R, Freedland KE, Clouse RE, Lustman PJ. Association of depression and diabetes complications: a meta-analysis. Psychosom Med. 2001;63(4):619–30.
5. Black SA, Markides KS, Ray LA. Depression predicts increased incidence of adverse health outcomes in older Mexican Americans with type 2 diabetes. Diabetes Care. 2003;26(10):2822–8.
6. Egede LE, Nietert PJ, Zheng D. Depression and all-cause and coronary heart disease mortality among adults with and without diabetes. Diabetes Care. 2005;28(6):1339–45.
7. Lin EH, Rutter CM, Katon W, Heckbert SR, Ciechanowski P, Oliver MM, et al. Depression and advanced complications of diabetes: a prospective cohort study. Diabetes Care. 2010;33(2):264–9.
8. Sieu N, Katon W, Lin EH, Russo J, Ludman E, Ciechanowski P. Depression and incident diabetic retinopathy: a prospective cohort study. Gen Hosp Psychiatry. 2011;33(5):429–35.
9. Williams LH, Rutter CM, Katon WJ, Reiber GE, Ciechanowski P, Heckbert SR, et al. Depression and incident diabetic foot ulcers: a prospective cohort study. Am J Med. 2010;123(8):748–54 e3.
10. Gonzalez JS, Vileikyte L, Ulbrecht JS, Rubin RR, Garrow AP, Delgado C, et al. Depression predicts first but not recurrent diabetic foot ulcers. Diabetologia. 2010;53(10):2241–8.
11. Katon WJ, Lin EH, Williams LH, Ciechanowski P, Heckbert SR, Ludman E, et al. Comorbid depression is associated with an increased risk of dementia diagnosis in patients with diabetes: a prospective cohort study. J Gen Intern Med. 2010;25(5):423–9.
12. Davydow DS, Russo JE, Ludman E, Ciechanowski P, Lin EH, Von Korff M, et al. The association of comorbid depression with intensive care unit admission in patients with diabetes: a prospective cohort study. Psychosomatics. 2011;52(2):117–26.
13. van Steenbergen-Weijenburg KM, van Puffelen AL, Horn EK, Nuyen J, van Dam PS, van Benthem TB, et al. More co-morbid depression in patients with type 2 diabetes with multiple complications. An observational study at a specialized outpatient clinic. Diabet Med. 2011; 28(1):86–9.
14. Vileikyte L, Peyrot M, Gonzalez JS, Rubin RR, Garrow AP, Stickings D, et al. Predictors of depressive symptoms in persons with diabetic peripheral neuropathy: a longitudinal study. Diabetologia. 2009;52(7):1265–73.
15. De Berardis G, Pellegrini F, Franciosi M, Belfiglio M, Di Nardo B, Greenfield S, et al. Identifying patients with type 2 diabetes with a higher likelihood of erectile dysfunction: the role of the interaction between clinical and psychological factors. J Urol. 2003;169(4):1422–8.

16. Lustman PJ, Penckofer SM, Clouse RE. Recent advances in understanding depression in adults with diabetes. Curr Diab Rep. 2007;7(2):114–22.
17. Golden SH. A review of the evidence for a neuroendocrine link between stress, depression and diabetes mellitus. Curr Diabetes Rev. 2007;3(4):252–9.
18. Lloyd CE, Pambianco G, Orchard TJ. Does diabetes-related distress explain the presence of depressive symptoms and/or poor self-care in individuals with type 1 diabetes? Diabet Med. 2010;27(2):234–7.
19. Gendelman N, Snell-Bergeon JK, McFann K, Kinney G, Paul Wadwa R, Bishop F, et al. Prevalence and correlates of depression in individuals with and without type 1 diabetes. Diabetes Care. 2009;32(4):575–9.
20. Fisher L, Skaff MM, Mullan JT, Arean P, Glasgow R, Masharani U. A longitudinal study of affective and anxiety disorders, depressive affect and diabetes distress in adults with type 2 diabetes. Diabet Med. 2008;25(9):1096–101.
21. Pouwer F, Skinner TC, Pibernik-Okanovic M, Beekman AT, Cradock S, Szabo S, et al. Serious diabetes-specific emotional problems and depression in a Croatian-Dutch-English survey from the European depression in diabetes [EDID] research consortium. Diabetes Res Clin Pract. 2005;70(2):166–73.
22. Fisher L, Skaff MM, Mullan JT, Arean P, Mohr D, Masharani U, et al. Clinical depression versus distress among patients with type 2 diabetes: not just a question of semantics. Diabetes Care. 2007;30(3):542–8.
23. Fisher L, Mullan JT, Arean P, Glasgow RE, Hessler D, Masharani U. Diabetes distress but not clinical depression or depressive symptoms is associated with glycemic control in both cross-sectional and longitudinal analyses. Diabetes Care. 2010;33(1):23–8.
24. Nouwen A, Ford T, Balan A, White DG. Illness intrusiveness and the longitudinal prediction of depression in adults with newly diagnosed type 2 diabetes mellitus. Diabetologia. 2011; 54(S1):390.
25. Snoek FJ, Hogenelst MH. Psychological implications of diabetes mellitus. Ned Tijdschr Geneeskd. 2008;152(44):2395–9.
26. Pouwer F, Tack CJ, Geelhoed-Duijvestijn PH, Bazelmans E, Beekman AT, Heine RJ, et al. Limited effect of screening for depression with written feedback in outpatients with diabetes mellitus: a randomised controlled trial. Diabetologia. 2011;54(4):741–8.
27. Pibernik-Okanović M, Ajduković D, Šekerija M, Poljak I, Hermanns N. Should we expect gender differences in reporting of depressive symptoms and seeking of professional help among diabetic patients? Diabetologia. 2011;54(Suppl1):S390.
28. Pibernik-Okanovic M, Ajdukovic D, Lovrencic M, Hermanns N. Does treatment of subsyndromal depression improve depression and diabetes related outcomes: protocol for a randomised controlled comparison of psycho-education, physical exercise and treatment as usual. Trials. 2011;12(1):17.
29. Arroll B, Goodyear-Smith F, Kerse N, Fishman T, Gunn J. Effect of the addition of a "help" question to two screening questions on specificity for diagnosis of depression in general practice: diagnostic validity study. BMJ. 2005;331(7521):884.
30. UK National Screening Committee. Criteria for appraising the viability, effectiveness and appropriateness of a screening programme [Internet] 2009 [Cited 2012 Feb]. www.screening.hhs.uk/criteria.
31. van der Feltz-Cornelis CM, Nuyen J, Stoop C, Chan J, Jacobson AM, Katon W, et al. Effect of interventions for major depressive disorder and significant depressive symptoms in patients with diabetes mellitus: a systematic review and meta-analysis. Gen Hosp Psychiatry. 2010; 32(4):380–95.
32. Katon WJ, Lin EH, Von Korff M. Ciechanowski P, Ludman EJ, Young B, et al. Collaborative care for patients with depression and chronic illnesses. N Engl J Med. 2010;363(27):2611–20.
33. Markowitz SM, Gonzalez JS, Wilkinson JL, Safren SA. A review of treating depression in diabetes: emerging findings. Psychosomatics. 2011;52(1):1–18.
34. Gonzalez JS, Safren SA, Cagliero E, Wexler DJ, Delahanty L, Wittenberg E, et al. Depression, self-care, and medication adherence in type 2 diabetes: relationships across the full range of symptom severity. Diabetes Care. 2007;30(9):2222–7.

35. Lorig K, Ritter PL, Villa F, Piette JD. Spanish diabetes self-management with and without automated telephone reinforcement: two randomized trials. Diabetes Care. 2008;31(3):408–14.
36. Carver CS. Affect and the functional bases of behavior: on the dimensional structure of affective experience. Pers Soc Psychol Rev. 2001;5(4):345–56.
37. Devins GM, Mendelssohn DC, Barre PE, Binik YM. Predialysis psychoeducational intervention and coping styles influence time to dialysis in chronic kidney disease. Am J Kidney Dis. 2003;42(4):693–703.
38. Gonzalez JS, Fisher L, Polonsky WH. Depression in diabetes: have we been missing something important? Diabetes Care. 2011;34(1):236–9.
39. Mead N, Bower P. Patient-centredness: a conceptual framework and review of the empirical literature. Soc Sci Med. 2000;51(7):1087–110.
40. Schulberg HC, Saul M, McClelland M, Ganguli M, Christy W, Frank R. Assessing depression in primary medical and psychiatric practices. Arch Gen Psychiatry. 1985;42(12):1164–70.
41. Lawlor DA, Hopker SW. The effectiveness of exercise as an intervention in the management of depression: systematic review and meta-regression analysis of randomised controlled trials. BMJ. 2001;322(7289):763–7.
42. Blumenthal JA, Babyak MA, Doraiswamy PM, Watkins L, Hoffman BM, Barbour KA, et al. Exercise and pharmacotherapy in the treatment of major depressive disorder. Psychosom Med. 2007;69(7):587–96.
43. Dowrick C, Dunn G, Ayuso-Mateos JL, Dalgard OS, Page H, Lehtinen V, et al. Problem solving treatment and group psychoeducation for depression: multicentre randomised controlled trial. BMJ. 2000;321(7274):1450.
44. Plack K, Herpertz S, Petrak F. Behavioral medicine interventions in diabetes. Curr Opin Psychiatry. 2010;23(2):131–8.
45. Norris SL, Engelgau MM, Venkat Narayan KM. Effectiveness of self-management training in type 2 diabetes. Diabetes Care. 2001;24(3):561–87.
46. Cochran J, Conn VS. Meta-analysis of quality of life outcomes following diabetes self-management training. Diabetes Educ. 2008;34(5):815–23.
47. Norris SL, Lau J, Smith SJ, Schmid CH, Engelgau MM. Self-management education for adults with type 2 diabetes. Diabetes Care. 2002;25(7):1159–71.
48. Cox DJ, Gonder-Frederick L, Polonsky W, Schlundt D, Kovatchev B, Clarke W. Blood glucose awareness training (BGAT-2). Diabetes Care. 2001;24(4):637–42.
49. Surwit RS, van Tilburg MAL, Zucker N, McCaskill CC, Parekh P, Feinglos MN, et al. Stress management improves long-term glycemic control in type 2 diabetes. Diabetes Care. 2002; 25(1):30–4.
50. Ayalon L, Goldfracht M, Bech P. 'Do you think you suffer from depression?' Reevaluating the use of a single item question for the screening of depression in older primary care patients. Int J Geriatr Psychiatry. 2010;25(5):497–502.
51. Peyrot M, Rubin RR. Behavioral and psychosocial interventions in diabetes: a conceptual review. Diabetes Care. 2007;30(10):2433–40.

Chapter 10
Measuring and Assessing Depression in People with Diabetes: Implications for Clinical Practice

Frans Pouwer and Evan Atlantis

Abstract Diabetes is an increasing global health and economic burden that is frequently associated with and worsened by clinically significant depression or anxiety. This chapter focuses on the history and evolution of the concept of depression and will also describe some of the uncertainties and controversy surrounding psychiatric nosology. Depression as a syndrome of pathological emotions should be diagnosed using operationalized criteria; however, at the same time, depression should not be reified as a discrete construct with absolute boundaries. Depression is often comorbid with anxiety and other mental disorders, which could be clinically important for diabetes. As with other medical syndromes, there is substantial heterogeneity between patients within psychiatric diagnostic groups. Clinically significant depression is defined using cutoff scores for self-rated symptoms using various psychometrics, which correlate reasonably well with operationalized diagnoses. Both methods classify persons into clinically significant dichotomies of depression for diabetes. This chapter considers the implications of these diagnoses for clinical practice and makes suggestions as to the way forward both in terms of the identification of people with comorbid depression and diabetes and for treatment and care. Computerized assessment, for example, with computerized adaptive testing (CAT), can facilitate time-efficient depression screening in busy clinic settings.

Keywords Depression • Anxiety • Screening • Diagnosis • Psychiatric nosology Diabetes

---

F. Pouwer, Ph.D.
Medical Psychology and Neuropsychology, Center of Research on Psychology in Somatic diseases (CoRPS) FSW, Tilburg University, Tilburg, The Netherlands

E. Atlantis, Ph.D. (✉)
Family & Community Health Research Group, School of Nursing and Midwifery, University of Western Sydney,
Locked Bag 1797, Penrith NSW 2751, Australia
e-mail: e.atlantis@uws.edu.au

C.E. Lloyd et al. (eds.), *Screening for Depression and Other Psychological Problems in Diabetes*,
DOI 10.1007/978-0-85729-751-8_10,

Introduction

The previous chapters in this book have emphasized that depression is common in people with diabetes, with the odds of having depression being at least twofold higher in those with either type 1 or type 2 diabetes, compared to those without this condition [1–3]. People with diabetes who also have complications are at a particularly increased risk for depression [4], and depressed patients with diabetes are more likely to be in poor glycemic control [5]. Current systematic reviews of prospective cohort studies have shown that the association between type 2 diabetes and depression is bidirectional, though the risk of type 2 diabetes associated with depression might be higher than the risk in the reverse direction [6, 7].

There is substantial heterogeneity between type 1 and type 2 diabetes comorbidity with depression, which is partly explained by their different etiologies [8]. Type 1 diabetes results from a cellular-mediated autoimmune destruction of the pancreatic β-cells that usually develops in childhood and adolescence, and therefore is likely to be a significant predictor of depression rather than the reverse. Type 2 diabetes, which usually appears in adulthood, occurs through a combination of insulin resistance and pancreatic β-cell dysfunction. Hyperglycemia develops gradually as a result of progressive β-cell dysfunction. Obesity, poor diet, and physical inactivity are important risk factors for the development of diabetes, factors which should also be assessed in patients with depression.

The excess health and economic burden of comorbid depression is found uniformly in both people with type 1 and type 2 diabetes. For instance, depression has been shown to have a negative effect on self-care behavior [9] and glycemic control [10], which is equivalent for both type 1 and type 2 diabetes. In addition, depression in people with type 1 or type 2 diabetes is frequently associated with low health-related quality of life scores [11–13], increased vascular events [14], cardiovascular disease mortality [15], and health service utilization and costs [16–18].

It is important to note that depression is often comorbid with anxiety disorders [19], which also could be pathological for diabetes. Like depression, clinically significant anxiety is common in people with diabetes [20] and has been shown to increase the risk of developing type 2 diabetes [21, 22]. Collectively, the existing evidence indicates that routine screening for depression, anxiety, or psychological distress in clinical practice could provide important information for diabetes treatment and prevention planning.

This chapter focuses on the different ways depression has been measured in scientific research and the implications this has for clinical practice. Nowadays, depression is often measured or assessed either by means of self-report measures or by means of a structured, psychiatric diagnostic interview. Diagnostic criteria of many diseases, including type 2 diabetes and depression, change over time, and it is important for both researchers and clinicians to understand the history of the concept of "depression." In this chapter, we will not only describe the different ways depression currently has been defined in the widely used international disease classification systems such as the *Diagnostic and Statistical Manual of Mental*

Disorders (*DSM*) and the *International Classification of Diseases* (*ICD*) but also highlight the changes that are to be expected for the new edition, the DSM-V. In addition, we consider how different tools have been used to quantify depression in research and the implications this has for clinical practice. Finally, several practical findings from the literature, related to depression assessment in diabetes, will be discussed. In research, for example, computerized versions of self-report measures have been compared with their paper-and-pencil versions, and computerized assessments have been evaluated in clinical care.

Nosology of Depression

Researchers and clinicians have been struggling for centuries to improve their knowledge about "depression" and of course to find better ways to improve treatment options for patients with depression. Currently, depression is considered to be a syndrome of pathological emotions diagnosed using operationalized criteria (DSM or ICD). Depression is usually measured or assessed either by means of self-report measures or by means of a structured, psychiatric diagnostic interview. Clinically significant depression is defined using cutoff scores (on a continuum of severity) for self-rated symptoms derived from a number of psychometrics (questionnaires), which correlate reasonably well with a formal diagnosis. Both methods classify persons into clinically significant dichotomies of depression for diabetes.

Depression: The History of an Important Construct

The ancient Greeks already described depression or depressed mood as a disease but did not distinguish it from other forms of mental illness. At that time, the general notion was that diseases were caused by an imbalance in four basic bodily fluids (blood, yellow bile, black bile, and phlegm). Interestingly, the word melancholia stems from the ancient Greek words melas, "black," and kholé, "bile." In his aphorisms, Hippocrates described melancholia as a disease caused by an excess of black bile [23]. Hippocrates has described a distinct disease pattern with particular mental and physical symptoms: "If a fright or loss of hope/depression (despondency) lasts for a long time, it is a melancholic affection." Aretaeus of Cappadocia also gave early descriptions of several diseases. He described and named diabetes, for example, and wrote: "Diabetes is a wonderful affection, not very frequent among men, being a melting down of the flesh and limbs into urine" [24]. Aretaeus also described that persons who suffered from melancholia were dull or stern, dejected or unreasonably inactive, lethargic, without any manifest cause [25]. It is important to note that the construct of melancholia was a broader concept than today's depression. Melancholia consisted of a symptom-cluster sadness, dejection, and hopelessness and sad mood and also included fears and anger. Until the seventeenth and eighteenth century, many Europeans used the word "melancholia" to describe a whole range of mental illnesses. The term "depression" that is being used nowadays stems from the Latin verb "deprimere," which means "to press down."

Depression: Modern Definitions in the Twentieth Century

For a very long period, there were many different definitions for psychiatric diseases. There was little agreement on which symptoms should be included, and this hampered effective communication between health care providers, researchers, and patients. Poor diagnostic criteria also slow down progress in scientific research, as results of studies are difficult to replicate or to compare with other scientific investigations. In response to these problems, the *Diagnostic and Statistical Manual of Mental Disorders*, First Edition (DSM-I) was published in 1952 [26]. This manual was prepared by the Committee on Nomenclature and Statistics of the American Psychiatric Association and contained the "depressive reaction." A few years earlier, in 1948, the World Health Organization (WHO) had published a new edition of the *Manual of the International Classification of Diseases, Injuries and Causes of Death* (*ICD-6*). Interestingly, in this new edition, the WHO had added a mental disorders section for the first time.

A new edition of the US manual, the DSM-II (published 1968), gave a new name to depression [27]. In this second edition, the term "depressive neurosis" was used as an "excessive reaction to internal conflict or an identifiable event." Both DSM-I and DSM-II were still strongly influenced by the psychodynamic theories. In the 1960s, the psychiatric disorders were generally divided into two groups: (1) disorders in which a disturbance in mental functioning was the result from or was precipitated by a primary impairment of the function of the brain, generally caused by diffuse impairment of brain tissue, and (2) disorders which were the result of a more general difficulty of the individual in adapting to certain environmental events. Any associated brain function disturbance was secondary to the psychiatric disorder.

Introduction of a New Term: "Major Depressive Disorder"

The term "major depressive disorder," still in use nowadays, was first described in the 1970s. At that time, new proposals were made for diagnostic criteria that were based on research regarding different patterns of symptoms. Important work has been done by Feighner and colleagues [28] and later by Spitzer and Robins [29]. Published in 1972, the Feighner criteria were soon widely used in research, and these criteria formed the basis for the development of the Research Diagnostic Criteria, which in turn were central to the development of DSM-III [30, 31]. The Feighner criteria were important in that they proposed to make systematic use of operationalized diagnostic criteria. These criteria also emphasized illness course and outcome. Last but certainly not least, they also emphasized the need to base psychiatric diagnostic criteria on empirical evidence as much as possible [30].

The definition of major depression was first incorporated into the DSM-III [31]. In this third version of the DSM, the older terms "depressive reaction" and "neurotic depression" were eliminated. The DSM-III and also DSM-IV are much more research-based. A diagnosis of a depressive disorder in both DSM-IV and ICD-10 requires a major disturbance in mood, i.e., "depressed mood" or "loss of interest or pleasure." These classification systems do not use a clear etiology (e.g., certain biochemical processes) or use the response to treatment or outcome as an important factor in the classification of a mood disorder. For a diagnosis of a mood disorder, both ICD-10 and DSM-IV have eight symptoms in common: depressed mood, loss of interest, decrease in energy or increased fatigue, sleep disturbance, appetite disturbance, recurrent thoughts of death, inability to concentrate or indecisiveness, and psychomotor agitation or retardation. The ICD-10, however, has two additional items: reduced self-esteem or reduced self-confidence and ideas of guilt and unworthiness, where the DSM-IV combines inappropriate and/or excessive guilt with feelings of worthlessness.

The ancient term "melancholia" that originates from the Greek words for "black bile" (melas kholé) still survives in the melancholic subtype in the DSM-IV-TR, published in 2000 [32]. Symptoms of melancholic depression are currently anhedonia, which is the inability to find pleasure in positive things, or lack of mood reactivity (i.e., mood does not improve in response to positive events) and at least three of: depression that is subjectively different from grief or loss, severe weight loss or loss of appetite, psychomotor agitation or retardation, early morning awakening, guilt that is excessive, and worse mood in the morning.

Heterogeneity of Depression

Although patients may be diagnosed with the same mood disorder, for example, a major depressive disorder, their symptoms can vary. For example, the criterion "disturbed sleep" can mean that patients suffer from hypersomnia but also insomnia. The same holds true for "disturbed eating," as both a marked decrease and an obvious increase in appetite (and as a result also of weight loss and weight gain) are symptoms of depression. Moreover, both psychomotor agitation and psychomotor retardation are symptoms of major depressive disorder. Thus, it is likely that there are "different depressions."

Different tools can be used to measure subdimensions of depression, such as anhedonia, somatic symptoms of depression, cognitive symptoms of depression, atypical depression, and melancholic depression. For example, with the second version of the Beck Depression Inventory (BDI-II, a widely used depression questionnaire), two different dimensions can be calculated: the cognitive-affective component (e.g., mood) and the physical or somatic component (e.g., loss of appetite). The affective subscale of the BDI-II contains eight items: past failures, pessimism, guilt feelings, punishment feelings, self-dislike, self-criticalness, suicidal thoughts or wishes, and worthlessness. The somatic subscale consists of the other thirteen items: sadness, loss of pleasure, crying, agitation, loss of interest, indecisiveness, loss of energy, change in sleep patterns, irritability, change in appetite, concentration difficulties, tiredness and/or fatigue, and loss of interest in sex. The use of these subscales and the symptoms therein may well be important, when making treatment decisions but also in teasing out their relative importance in the etiology of disease. For example, Poole and colleagues [33] describe in their review that in patients with post-acute coronary syndrome, particularly the somatic symptoms of depression appear to be more "cardiotoxic" than the cognitive depression symptoms. Furthermore, they describe that depression following an acute coronary syndrome generally does not respond to antidepressant medication. The results of a study by Poole et al. [33] suggest that the type of depression that develops after a myocardial infarction may have a different, inflammation-based etiology than depression in the general population. The question then arises: "should we use different tools for diagnosing depression with a dominance of somatic symptoms or a dominance of cognitive symptoms, or perhaps both?" The answer is probably given in a commentary to the review of Poole et al., by Peter de Jonge [34], who wrote: "I believe that Poole et al. are teaching us a valuable lesson that goes beyond the field of cardiopsychiatry and psychosomatic research. Only the future can tell whether the identification of inflammation-based depression will be truly influential" [34]. This fascinating puzzle has yet to be solved, but there is a growing body of evidence based on cross-sectional studies which suggests that the assessment of somatic symptoms, resulting in sympathetic nervous system hyperactivity, might be more clinically useful than cognitive symptoms for diabetes [35, 36].

It is expected that in 2013, the new DSM-V will be published. According to the website of the DSM-V, the definition of major depression will not change considerably in the DSM-V (www.dsm5.org/Pages/Default.aspx). Interestingly, a new category will be added, "mixed depression and anxiety." In this category, the patient has three or four symptoms of a major depression (including depressed, anhedonia), but these symptoms are accompanied by anxious distress (e.g., irrational worry, having trouble relaxing, motor tension, preoccupation with unpleasant worries or fear that something awful may happen). The implications for care as the new criteria are put into practice remain to be seen.

Selecting a Depression Questionnaire for Use in Clinical Diabetes Care

Health care providers who want to measure depression in their patients are faced with a difficult task, as they can choose from a large number of validated depression questionnaires that have been developed in the past decades. Roy and colleagues [37] have published a systematic review of depression screening tools that are currently being used in diabetes research. Of the 234 studies reviewed, it appeared that the BDI (24%), the Center for Epidemiologic Studies Depression Scale (CES-D, 21%), and the PHQ-9 (Patient Health Questionnaire, 11%) were the most commonly used depression questionnaires in diabetes research. Depression screening questionnaires can be divided into two groups: (1) depression questionnaires that invite the patient to rate the severity or frequency of various symptoms that are not necessarily included in the definition of major depression and (2) symptom count questionnaires that are based on the diagnostic criteria for depression. The BDI and the CES-D are good examples of instruments that are based on frequency of various symptoms, whereas the PHQ-9 is a good example of a symptom count questionnaire that is based on the DSM-IV criteria. It is important to emphasize that both types of depression questionnaires are screening tools and should not be used for a clinical diagnosis. Even the self-report measures that use the diagnostic criteria of the DSM-IV, such as the PHQ-9, should be used with caution and regarded as a first step toward a more definite diagnosis. The presence of clinically significant depression warrants further clinical assessment for depression. A diagnosis of a mental disorder can only be made using a structured psychiatric diagnostic interview.

An important feature of an instrument that will be used in a busy clinical practice is its feasibility or ease of administration. The BDI consists of 21 items, the CES-D of 20 items, and the PHQ-9 of only 9 items. Shorter questionnaires are available. For example, the WHO-5, recommended for use in the Global Guidelines for Type 2 Diabetes (section 4, psychosocial guidelines), by the World Health Organization, consists of only five positively worded items [38]. Another important characteristic of a good screening tool is its ability to recognize patients with depression and those without depression. Roy et al. [37] concluded that, given the limited data available and the lack of any published comparisons between questionnaires, it is not possible yet to conclude which of these have the best screening performance (in terms of sensitivity and specificity).

In summary, clinicians and researchers who wish to measure depression in patients with diabetes can choose from a large number of validated depression questionnaires. The most widely used depression measures in diabetes are the BDI, the CES-D, and the PHQ-9. These questionnaires are reliable and valid tools to assess clinically significant symptoms of depression, but it is still unclear which instrument has the best psychometric properties in patients with diabetes, as most validation work has been conducted in large nondiabetic groups.

Computerized Assessment

For several questionnaires, computerized versions have been developed, and these have several advantages. For example, some patients prefer to reveal some types of very personal information to a computer instead of a person. Furthermore, the calculation of the subscales and the comparison with normal scores are quicker and much less susceptible to mistakes if they are conducted by a personal computer, compared to humans. Total scores can automatically be stored in the patient files.

The instructions can be given by the computer, and the scores of the patient can also be printed, along with an interpretation of the score. It seems important that the assessment of depression is done in a relatively short time. A recent study by Valenstein et al. concluded that screening for depression would not meet the reasonable criteria for cost utility if the cost of administering a single test was substantially higher than five US dollar, where that cost comprised a fee for the instrument use, 6 min of staff time, and 1 min of physician time [39]. Earlier research in a group of 76 outpatients with diabetes has shown that a computerized version of the Well-Being Questionnaire (WBQ) was equivalent to the paper-and-pencil version [40]. The scales showed high test-retest correlations, and the means, dispersions, kurtosis, and skewness were found to be approximately the same in both versions. Almost all subjects reported that using the personal computer to complete a questionnaire was easy to do [40]. The authors concluded that the paper-and-pencil and the computerized versions of the WBQ and DTSQ can be considered equivalent. Therefore, the norms and cutoff scores obtained from paper-and-pencil assessments can be used in computerized versions of the WBQ and DTSQ and vice versa [40].

Other developments can facilitate the assessment of depression in patients with diabetes. For example, if using the internet, patients can complete the questionnaires at home. Besides, online treatment for depression, based on the principles of cognitive behavioral therapy, appears to be feasible and effective in reducing depressive symptoms in adults with type 1 and type 2 diabetes [41]. This intervention was also effective in patients with more severe depression and also reduced the level of diabetes-specific emotional distress in depressed patients [41, 42]. What is also important is that new computerized assessment techniques have been developed that make use of computerized adaptive testing (CAT). CAT is a term used to describe a technology for interactive administration of tests that adjusts the test to the scores of the patient. Such tests are adaptive because the testing is driven by an algorithm that selects new questions in a fraction of a second in response to the answers of the patients. At each step, the patient's earlier responses determine whether the computer will ask another question and also which question. The test stops if the depression score has been estimated at a certain level of precision. The number of questions is therefore often lower. Gardner and colleagues [43] studied a computerized adaptive testing version of the Beck Depression Inventory and concluded that using CAT techniques, this instrument could be "converted to a far more efficient adaptive test without loss of accuracy." In sum, computerized assessment and computerized adaptive testing of depression are recommendable as they can save time and reduce errors.

Is Depression the Only Relevant Construct to Assess?

Of all the emotional problems that can occur in patients with diabetes, depression has received the most attention of researchers. A potential consequence is that the focus may be too much toward depression. As discussed in earlier chapters, other important emotional complaints such as anxiety or diabetes-specific emotional distress can be overlooked. It may be relevant for clinicians to assess levels of anxiety and diabetes-specific emotional distress, as research has shown that depressed patients with diabetes often suffer from higher levels of anxiety and diabetes-specific emotional distress. A multicenter study from the European Depression in Diabetes Research Consortium combined data from the United Kingdom, Croatia, and the Netherlands and showed that diabetes patients had relatively high levels of diabetes-specific stress [44]. Patients with high levels of diabetes-specific emotional stress can suffer from fear of hypoglycemia, worries about complications, can experience uncomfortable interactions with other persons around diabetes, or experience a lack of support for health care providers or family [44].

Conclusions

Depression is a syndrome of pathological emotions diagnosed using operationalized criteria, with clinically significant depression defined using cutoff scores on a continuum of severity for self-rated symptoms using various psychometrics, which correlate reasonably well with a psychiatric diagnosis. As with other medical syndromes, there may be substantial heterogeneity between patients within diagnostic groups. Clinicians can use different subscales of depression questionnaires such as the BDI if they wish to assess subdimensions of depression, given that somatic symptoms might be more clinically useful than cognitive symptoms for diabetes. A further important issue to consider is that depression is often comorbid with anxiety and other mental disorders, which could be clinically important for diabetes. Computerized assessment, for example, with computerized adaptive testing (CAT), can facilitate time-efficient assessments in busy clinics.

References

1. Ali S, Stone MA, Peters JL, Davies MJ, Khunti K. The prevalence of co-morbid depression in adults with type 2 diabetes: a systematic review and meta-analysis. Diabet Med. 2006;23(11):1165–73.
2. Barnard KD, Skinner TC, Peveler R. The prevalence of co-morbid depression in adults with type 1 diabetes: systematic literature review. Diabet Med. 2006;23(4):445–8.
3. Pouwer F, Geelhoed-Duijvestijn PH, Tack CJ, Bazelmans E, Beekman AJ, Heine RJ, et al. Prevalence of comorbid depression is high in out-patients with type 1 or type 2 diabetes mellitus. Results from three out-patient clinics in the Netherlands. Diabet Med. 2010;27:217–24.
4. de Groot M, Anderson R, Freedland KE, Clouse RE, Lustman PJ. Association of depression and diabetes complications: a meta-analysis. Psychosom Med. 2001;63(4):619–30.
5. Lustman PJ, Clouse RE. Depression in diabetic patients: the relationship between mood and glycemic control. J Diabetes Complications. 2005;19(2):113–22.
6. Mezuk B, Eaton WW, Albrecht S, Golden SH. Depression and type 2 diabetes over the lifespan: a meta-analysis. Diabetes Care. 2008;31(12):2383–90.

7. Nouwen A, Winkley K, Twisk J, Lloyd CE, Peyrot M, Ismail K, et al. European depression in diabetes (EDID) research consortium. Type 2 diabetes mellitus as a risk factor for the onset of depression: a systematic review and meta-analysis. Diabetologia. 2010;53(12):2480–6.
8. American Diabetes Association. Economic costs of diabetes in the U.S. In 2007. Diabetes Care. 2008;31:596–615.
9. Gonzalez JS, Peyrot M, McCarl LA, Collins EM, Serpa L, Mimiaga MJ, et al. Depression and diabetes treatment nonadherence: a meta-analysis. Diabetes Care. 2008;31:2398–403.
10. Lustman PJ, Anderson RJ, Freedland KE, de Groot M, Carney RM, Clouse RE. Depression and poor glycemic control: a meta-analytic review of the literature. Diabetes Care. 2000;23:934–42.
11. Atlantis E, Goldney RD, Eckert KA, Taylor AW, Phillips P. Trends in health-related quality of life and health service use associated with comorbid diabetes and major depression in South Australia, 1998–2008. Soc Psychiatry Psychiatr Epidemiol. 2012;47(6):871–7.
12. Hilliard ME, Herzer M, Dolan LM, Hood KK. Psychological screening in adolescents with type 1 diabetes predicts outcomes one year later. Diabetes Res Clin Pract. 2011;94(1):39–44.
13. Schram MT, Baan CA, Pouwer F. Depression and quality of life in patients with diabetes: a systematic review from the European depression in diabetes (EDID) research consortium. Curr Diabetes Rev. 2009;5(2):112–9.
14. Lin EH, Rutter CM, Katon W, Heckbert SR, Ciechanowski P, Oliver MM, et al. Depression and advanced complications of diabetes: a prospective cohort study. Diabetes Care. 2010;33:264–9.
15. Atlantis E, Shi Z, Penninx BJ, Wittert GA, Taylor A, Almeida OP. Chronic medical conditions mediate the association between depression and cardiovascular disease mortality. Soc Psychiatry Psychiatr Epidemiol. 2012;47(4):615–25. doi:10.1007/s00127–011–0365–9. Epub 2011 Mar 8.
16. Davydow DS, Russo JE, Ludman E, Ciechanowski P, Lin EH, Von Korff M, et al. The association of comorbid depression with intensive care unit admission in patients with diabetes: a prospective cohort study. Psychosomatics. 2011;52:117–26.
17. Hutter N, Schnurr A, Baumeister H. Healthcare costs in patients with diabetes mellitus and comorbid mental disorders – a systematic review. Diabetologia. 2010;53: 2470–2479. International Diabetes Federation. IDF diabetes atlas. 5th ed. Brussels: International Diabetes Federation; 2011.
18. Stewart SM, Rao U, Emslie GJ, Klein D, White PC. Depressive symptoms predict hospitalization for adolescents with type 1 diabetes mellitus. Pediatrics. 2005;115:1315–9.
19. Weich S, McBride O, Hussey D, Exeter D, Brugha T, McManus S. Latent class analysis of co-morbidity in the adult psychiatric morbidity survey in England 2007: implications for DSM-5 and ICD-11. Psychol Med. 2011;41(10):2201–12.
20. Li C, Barker L, Ford ES, Zhang X, Strine TW, Mokdad AH. Diabetes and anxiety in US adults: findings from the 2006 behavioral risk factor surveillance system. Diabet Med. 2008;25(7): 878–81.
21. Engum A. The role of depression and anxiety in onset of diabetes in a large population-based study. J Psychosom Res. 2007;62(1):31–8.
22. Eriksson AK, Ekbom A, Granath F, Hilding A, Efendic S, Ostenson CG. Psychological distress and risk of pre-diabetes and type 2 diabetes in a prospective study of Swedish middle-aged men and women. Diabet Med. 2008;25(7):834–42.
23. Hothersall D. Chapter 1: Psychology and the ancients. In: History of psychology. 4th ed. New York: Mc Graw-Hill; 2004. p. 15–32.
24. Clending L. Chapter 8: Aretaeus the Cappadocian. In: Source book of medical history. New York: Dover Publications; 1960. p. 52–7.
25. Adams F (trans). Chapter 5: Melancholy. In: The extant works of aretaeus, the cappadocian. Boston: Milford House Inc; 1972. p. 53–55.
26. American Psychiatric Association. Diagnostic and statistical manual: mental disorders. Washington: American Psychiatric Association; 1952.
27. American Psychiatric Association. Diagnostic and statistical manual of mental disorders. 2nd ed. Washington, DC: American Psychiatric Association; 1968.

28. Feighner JP, Robins E, Guze SB, Woodruff RA, Winokur G, Munoz R. Diagnostic criteria for use in psychiatric research. Arch Gen Psychiatry. 1972;26:57–63.
29. Spitzer RL, Robins E. Research diagnostic criteria: rationale and reliability. Arch Gen Psychiatry. 1978;35:773–82.
30. Kendler KS, Muñoz RA, Murphy G. The development of the feighner criteria: a historical perspective. Am J Psychiatry. 2010;167(2):134–42.
31. American Psychiatric Association. Diagnostic and statistical manual of mental disorders. 3rd ed. Washington, DC: American Psychiatric Association; 1980.
32. American Psychiatric Association. Diagnostic and statistical manual of mental disorders. 4th ed. Washington, DC: American Psychiatric Association; 2000, text revisions.
33. Poole L, Dickens C, Steptoe A. The puzzle of depression and acute coronary syndrome: reviewing the role of acute inflammation. J Psychosom Res. 2011;71(2):61–8.
34. de Jonge P. Depression deconstruction lessons from psychosomatic research. J Psychosom Res. 2011;71(2):59–60.
35. Licht CM, Vreeburg SA, van Reedt Dortland AK, Giltay EJ, Hoogendijk WJ, DeRijk RH, Vogelzangs N, Zitman FG, de Geus EJ, Penninx BW. Increased sympathetic and decreased parasympathetic activity rather than changes in hypothalamic-pituitary-adrenal axis activity is associated with metabolic abnormalities. J Clin Endocrinol Metab. 2010;95(5):2458–66.
36. Luppino FS, van Reedt Dortland AK, Wardenaar KJ, Bouvy PF, Giltay EJ, Zitman FG, Penninx BW. Symptom dimensions of depression and anxiety and the metabolic syndrome. Psychosom Med. 2011;73(3):257–64.
37. Roy T, Lloyd CE, Pouwer F, Holt RI, Sartorius N. Screening tools used for measuring depression among people with type 1 and type 2 diabetes: a systematic review. Diabet Med. 2012; 29(2):164–75.
38. IDF Clinical Guidelines Task Force. Global guideline for type 2 diabetes: recommendations for standard, comprehensive, and minimal care. Diabet Med. 2006;23(6):579–93.
39. Valenstein M, Vijan S, Zeber JE, Boehm K, Buttar A. The cost-utility of screening for depression in primary care. Ann Intern Med. 2001;134(5):345–60.
40. Pouwer F, Snoek FJ, van der Ploeg HM, Heine RJ, Brand AN. A comparison of the standard and the computerized versions of the well-being questionnaire (WBQ) and the diabetes treatment satisfaction questionnaire (DTSQ). Qual Life Res. 1998;7(1):33–8.
41. van Bastelaar KM, Pouwer F, Cuijpers P, Riper H, Snoek FJ. Web-based depression treatment for type 1 and type 2 diabetic patients: a randomized, controlled trial. Diabetes Care. 2011; 34(2):320–5.
42. van Bastelaar KM, Pouwer F, Cuijpers P, Riper H, Twisk JW, Snoek FJ. Is a severe clinical profile an effect modifier in a web-based depression treatment for adults with type 1 or type 2 diabetes? Secondary analyses from a randomized controlled trial. J Med Internet Res. 2012;14(1):e2.
43. Gardner W, Shear K, Kelleher KJ, Pajer KA, Mammen O, Buysse D, Frank E. Computerized adaptive measurement of depression: a simulation study. BMC Psychiatry. 2004;4:13.
44. Pouwer F, Skinner TC, Pibernik-Okanovic M, Beekman AT, Cradock S, Szabo S, Metelko Z, Snoek FJ. Serious diabetes-specific emotional problems and depression in a Croatian-Dutch-English survey from the European depression in diabetes [EDID] research consortium. Diabetes Res Clin Pract. 2005;70(2):166–73.

Index

C.E. Lloyd et al. (eds.), *Screening for Depression and Other Psychological Problems in Diabetes*,
DOI 10.1007/978-0-85729-751-8, © Springer-Verlag London 2013

P

Q

R